The Life and Times of a
Country Doctor

The Autobiography of James E. Albrecht, MD

I am indebted to you for
buying my book.

Thank you for sharing.

James W. Malatino

Published by:
James E. Albrecht, MD

distributed by:

j.e.a. enterprises
2487 Pleasant Valley Rd.
Jackson, WI 53037
414-677-2140

The author would consider it an honor to have any material in this book used for the betterment of humanity. Therefore, it is not necessary to ask for permission to use quotes from the book, but a note stating how you plan to use it would be appreciated.

First Printing, May 1993
Second Printing, June 1993
Printed and bound in the United States of America

Production by:
DeRaimo Publishing, Inc.
137 N. Main Street, West Bend, WI 53095
414/338-0651 • FAX: 414/338-4252

Table of Contents

Foreword

1

Dr. James Albrecht represents one member of a select group of physicians. Their practice experience spans the period of time from the traditional country doctor who made house calls carrying most of his medications and surgical instruments in a small black bag to today's era of modern medicine with its vast lists of pharmacologic miracles and dazzling array of computerized equipment. They have spanned the time when death from heart disease was considered natural to today's era of bypass surgeries, valve replacements and heart transplants.

If we have lost anything in all this progress, it is that we have lost the country doctor's personal approach. That special bond between the patient and the physician has been

1

replaced by a relationship between a consumer and a provider who is trying to preserve his "market share." I am dismayed by this change, and particularly by the onslaught of prepaid medical plans (HMOs and PPOs) that dictate which physician a patient may use. I once asked Dr. Albrecht his opinion of HMOs and PPOs. His well-put response was, "I have practiced medicine for over thirty years and have always been proud of the fact that people came to me because they liked me and thought I did a good job. But nowadays they come to me because my services are covered [by their insurance]."

Somehow, I hope we can find a blend between medical progress and the personal relationships we found so valuable and rewarding in the past era. Every new physician should have at his disposal the latest in medical technology. They should also have a measure of the compassion of Dr. James Albrecht.

Paul R. Rice, MD

2

It's quite a challenge and an honor to write about a physician who has been in practice since I was in first grade. With a great deal of humility, I have agreed to undertake the task.

Jim Albrecht, affectionately known to one and all as "Doc Albrecht," has practiced medicine in Jackson, Wisconsin for forty-five years. I have known him for the last eighteen of those years. Since 1983, "Doc" has been a partner of mine at the General Clinic. Although his office location has changed several times, Jim has never changed the way he practices medicine. Yes, he worked as hard as two doctors. But sometimes he seemed a paradox.

Jim could be caring and kind to his patients, and on the other hand could be firm, blunt and unyielding, particularly when he knew it was in their best interest. Jim's curiosity led him to try many new drugs and new techniques before they were generally accepted by other physicians, but at the same time, he clung to many of the old ways that seemed to work best and help his patients. He is a very kind, caring, and giving person, but a person who also has a great deal of pride in what he has accomplished. A contradiction to some, but a good physician to those who know him.

His autobiography reads well and tells us a great deal about the man and the times in which he practiced medicine. Those were certainly different times then now. Perhaps they were kinder and gentler. As I read Doc's story, I wish I could have practiced in Jackson, Wisconsin during the 1950s and 1960s. The story is entertaining and I think there are lessons in it for all of us.

I value Jim's continued association with the General Clinic and with me as a partner in the practice of medicine. I also value his friendship.

William J. Listwan, MD
President, General Clinic

3

More than fifty years ago my ministry as a Lutheran pastor began in a small congregation in Madison, Wisconsin, a city which is both the state capitol and the home of the chief state university. Some of the students at that university worshipped in that congregation, Bethel Lutheran Church. Among those students was a young man from Beaver Dam, Wisconsin who was enrolled in the medical college of that university. He and I became good friends. His name was James Albrecht.

He was then, and has remained throughout his life, dedicated to his craft as a doctor of medicine and has chosen to serve a rural community near where he was born and raised. His four decades of commitment to his type of service is both unusual and remarkable. It is an exciting record.

So is this volume, *Life and Times of a Country Doctor*, which describes what one dedicated person can mean to the welfare of the people with whom he has chosen to live. It is a heartwarming and exciting story.

Morris Wee

4

When I think of compassionate, principled and courageous people I have known through the years, Dr. Albrecht heads the list. Although he was always extremely busy doctoring, he was also interested in his great family and in social issues and social justice.

Thirty-five years ago my husband Bob Cross and I arrived in West Bend. Bob had just been hired to teach biology at West Bend High School. Another young biology teacher, Bob Larsen, was hired the same year.

The community was lovely, the citizens great, but the old Badger High School biology course was pretty outdated. The textbooks were old and the labs lacked necessary equipment.

The two Bobs made do, mildly complaining for a few years, but then asked for and were granted new textbooks. They worked through the summer on lesson plans and laboratory exercises. When the books arrived shortly before the opening of school, the new district superintendent examined the chapter on human biology, which had never before been taught in the community, and told the biology teachers "to pack them up and send them back."

Frustrated and looking for options, my husband contacted Dr. Albrecht and explained the situation. Doc said, "Bring me a few copies of the book and I'll see what I can do."

A few hours after receiving the books, he called to say that it was a much needed textbook. He took copies to the hospital for other doctors to examine. He also asked ministers and priests for their input.

Within the week, my husband and Bob Larsen received an unexpected call from the superintendent, who said the books could stay. The teachers were grateful to Dr. Albrecht.

Years ago there was a decision made that the newly formed AA group could no longer meet at Doc's church. Some church members felt that "those people" were not the kind of people that should be using the church's facilities — besides, they smoked!

When Dr. Albrecht heard about the decision to exclude the group, he went before the church council and told them that "if my friends are not welcome here, I guess I'm not welcome either."

The group was allowed to continue meeting at the church.

I am proud to count Doc Albrecht among my friends. Through this book, I'm sure you, too, will come to enjoy the pleasure of his company.

Hope Nelson

5

It is indeed an honor to be asked to write a foreword for Doc Albrecht's *Life and Times of a Country Doctor*. James E. Albrecht, MD, is the epitome of a family doctor, hired more than forty years ago to be "the doctor" for the village of Jackson. He has been a friend to the community ever since he arrived, at an annual salary of $2,500.

He has served his patients well as a very able physician, a friend and an employer. Doc Albrecht's main concern now, as it always has been, is for the welfare of his patients. Nothing is more important to Doc than making sure that his patients are well cared for.

He has been instrumental in the workings of his church. A permanent fixture in any village activity, such as the Fourth of July parade, the Founders Day parade, and a permanent member of the Businessmen's Club. The Doc has been completely committed to improving his community, as well as the lives of all of the people he touches.

Up until the time he merged with the larger General Clinic of West Bend, Doc was the second largest employer in the Village of Jackson. His office ran like clockwork out of his two-story house, which housed the medical laboratory. He had the world's most loyal employees because he was the most loyal employer.

To this day, with God looking over his shoulder, Doc is still actively involved in the practice of medicine by seeing as many patients as is humanly possible at his office in Jackson. He has given up hospital practice, but is still surprising his colleagues in the medical community with his medical manipulative arts.

I know you will enjoy reading the *Life and Times of a Country Doctor*, because this is an accurate reflection of Doc's memories of his hard times and good times in the medical community.

John R. Miller

6

One of Jesus' most vivid stories depicts the day of judgement when all the nations are gathered before the Lord and he separates the people as a shepherd separates the sheep from the goats. The dividing line is described in Matthew 25 as a series of simple actions: "I was hungry and you gave me food, I was thirsty and you gave me something to drink, I was a stranger and you welcomed me, I was naked and you gave me clothing, I was sick and you took care of me, I was in prison and you visited me."

Those on the left and the right, the "goats" and the "sheep," did not remember having had the opportunity to take action-in response to Jesus' need. "And when was it that we saw you sick or in prison and visited you?" they asked. (Sometimes our benevolence, or lack of it, escapes even our own notice.)

So Jesus made it clear: "Truly I tell you, just as you did it to one of the least of these who are members of my family, you did it to me."

Lutheran Social Services is privileged to have in James Albrecht a friend whose faith springs to action. Among his friends are those who some might consider "the least" within the human family: mothers and babies from problem pregnancies, teens and adults struggling with addictions, men and women who are both poor and sick. We are honored that Doc Albrecht has chosen to direct the proceeds of this book toward our efforts to help people improve the quality of their lives. He has created something as unique as his own remarkable journey. *The Life and Times of a Country Doctor* inspires, informs, and entertains, but even more, it provides welcome and care and nourishment to some new friends of the good doctor.

Robert E. Duea, president and CEO
Lutheran Social Services
of Wisconsin and Upper Michigan

Acknowledgements

While the title "Into Life Eternal" might be better termed an epilogue, I feel it fitting to place it at the beginning rather than the end of this book. Marian shared my life for forty-eight of my seventy-seven years. She had a more profound influence in shaping my life than any other human. After two and one half months of reflection, I still feel it appropriate that this autobiography should be dedicated to her memory, to the Glory of God and to the fellowship of believers, whoever they may be.

I acknowledge with appreciation the love and support of my family, Lynn Vegafria, Peter Albrecht, Dr. Charles Albrecht, as well as my grandchildren, David and Cora Vegafria. May their lives be as filled with the love of God and the caring love and fellowship of those they come in contact with as Marian and I enjoyed.

I acknowledge with appreciation the support of my colleagues and staff of the General Clinic, both at the main office in West Bend and our Jackson office.

A special note of thanks to those long-time employees of the Jackson Medical Service from the start of my practice in 1948, with apologies to those I have neglected to mention by name, as Marian and I attempted to remember all those to whom we are indebted.

Some of those employees who transferred to the General Clinic when the Jackson Medical Service merged in 1983 have put up with me for a long time. This year, Dolores Mayer will have been with me twenty-five years and has been of invaluable service. Other current employees of the General Clinic sharing experiences when I was the "Chief" instead of just one of the Indians include Kay Chantelois, MaryAnn Ziemann, Debbie Racette, Nancy Gumm, and Dr. Sandra Byerly. I thank them as well as all others who have helped, working together as a team, to accomplish what God would have us do.

Very special thanks are due to my friends John Miller, who followed in his father's footsteps as a member of the professional management team, Gardner and Miller, and Sue Calhoun, a long-time friend and secretarial employee who still comes to my home, with no recompense, to help me keep my records straight as she did when she was my employee.

Without the challenge of a postcard from Muriel Kroening, the verbal encouragement of Marty Silseth of Lutheran Social Services, and the written encouragement in a letter a week later from John Puotinen, Director of Planned Giving of Lutheran Social Services — all prompting me to write The Life and Times of A Country Doctor — this book would probably not have been written. Those pieces of advice seemed more than coincidence and I perceived it as a nonverbal prodding by God to get to work: May He find the effort acceptable and may it accomplish whatever purpose He had in mind.

All proceeds from this, the story of my life, after initial costs have been amortized, will be dedicated to ongoing support of the work of Lutheran Social Services as a living memorial to both Marian and me.

For the encouragement of the officers and administration of the General Clinic, and support of all the employees, I am grateful.

In particular, I would like to acknowledge the invaluable assistance of Jane Grady who did the transcription of my original dictation. My wife Marian edited the first seventeen chapters. My daughter Lynn and I have had the professional assistance of Frank DeRaimo, Allan Price, and David Rank, with the supporting cast of all the employees of DeRaimo Publishing, Inc. I appreciate the friendship and cooperation I enjoy as we jointly work together to accomplish the purpose intended.

Early encouragement and suggestions from my friend Richard Kellow and his ongoing support are appreciated, as is the contribution of his daughter-in-law, attorney Linda Kellow, as she, together with my friend, John Miller, do the work in my stead to accomplish the settlement of Marian's estate. (This demonstrates that I practice what I preach. I think I would mess things up more trying to do the work they have been trained to do than if they tried to practice medicine without a license.)

I appreciate Jim Spella, my attorney, who has given me both professional and emotional support over many years. He currently is helping in the ongoing role of making this book and the related projects of Painter and Potter successful. These projects include the production and distribution of the prints of several of Marian's paintings together with notepaper, incorporating four of our favorite paintings. These projects, too, are designed to support God's work through the Washington

County Historical Society and the Crossways Lutheran Camping Ministries organizations, as well as other charitable causes.

A very special thanks to my friends Steve Niebauer and his wife Nancy for their offer, gratefully accepted, to work with me, at no recompense, in locally distributing my book, the prints of Marian's paintings and the notepaper through their pharmacies, to enhance the charitable course we have embarked on.

(It has been said, "Chickens come home to roost." Forty years ago, Steve's father, Jim Niebauer and Carl Kircher accepted my invitation to open a pharmacy in my office at Jackson to enable me to become the first nondispensing physician in Washington County. Our agreeable relationship over the years has been mutually advantageous and deeply appreciated.)

To all others, whether mentioned in my autobiography or not, who have been of help in stimulating my visions and achieving my dream, I give my thanks. Most especially do I appreciate the love and support of the many individuals over three generations I have been privileged to serve as a physician and friend.

To my readers, I hope you find this story of my life a good investment of your time and dollars.

May you all enjoy the fullness of life and the same sense of fellowship with God and your contemporaries as Marian and I have enjoyed.

Your Friend,
James Albrecht, MD

* * * * *

Postcard sent to me by M.N. Kroening, postmark July 31, 1992:
Dear Doc —
I got to thinking about the story you told me about snow-

shoeing in to treat the little girl who got burned during a blizzard in an isolated farmhouse. PLEASE Doc, WRITE A BOOK. "The Life & Times of a Country Doctor." If you just told all your tales into a recorder and let someone transcribe it for you, it would be a fascinating story. Add a chapter of biography. Bestseller Material. Don't just think about it, DO IT. Please?
Muriel Kroenig

* * * * *

Letter from Lutheran Social Services, dated July 22, 1992:

Dear Dr. Albrecht:

Thank you for the opportunity to meet you and to enjoy good conversation and good food with you and Marty Silseth last Tuesday noon. I concur with Marty's belief that you should write a book about your life story! I was fascinated and inspired by the experience you shared, and would have enjoyed more time for discussion.

Please know that we value your friendship with Lutheran Social Services, and that your partnership with us serves the needs of many people who come to LSS for help.

I look forward to seeing you again, and pray for God's continuing blessing upon you and your family.

Sincerely,
Pastor John V. Puotinen
Director
Planned Giving and Major Gifts

Prologue
Into Life
Eternal
(Originally written for
the funeral of
Marian Albrecht,
December 12, 1992.)

T he early morning of December 8, 1992, was the
first day of my life as a widower. Marian, my partner of forty-eight years, died the previous night at 8:30 after
a fifty-two-hour battle with death following a stroke at 5:15
on December 5, 1992.

Her editing of the story of my life ends with the seventeenth
chapter. The remainder of the book will be edited by others.
My autobiography will be dedicated to her memory, to the Glory
of God and to the fellowship of believers whoever they may
be.

The Fifth Avenue United Methodist Church of West Bend
had invited us to participate in their annual Bethlehem Journey
on Friday night and Saturday afternoon. Marian played the
zither in King Herod's Court while I was demonstrating on the

13

potter's wheel downstairs. It was for her a culmination of a lifetime of service in the Kingdom of God.

As we were going home, discussing with appreciation the events of the day and looking forward to getting ready to go to a Christmas party of the Jackson Business Association, little did we know that within one-half hour the final chapter of her life would begin. She proceeded to wrap a painting we planned to give as a door prize, while I was to unpack my pottery supplies from the station wagon, bearing the license plate "WE NJOY." As I came in with the second load, I heard a noise downstairs, found her comatose on the floor and realized she had suffered a stroke. The picture she had wrapped had fallen to one side. After getting her into a position of relative comfort and trying to give her some orange juice, I dialed 911.

Within a few minutes, the rescue squad arrived to convey her to St. Joseph's Community Hospital in West Bend where my medical colleagues, nursing and ancillary staff provided loving care, of which she was unaware, as her body put on the age-old battle to survive the departure of the spirit. There was little doubt of the ultimate outcome. The die was cast. The prognosis grave. While she had survived numerous other seemingly catastrophic problems over many years, five in the last six years, this was to be the beginning of the end of her earthly journey. When it became apparent that it was only a matter of time, the children and I requested that her living will be honored and she was allowed to expire over the next ten hours.

During that ten hours of reflection and introspection, I was reminded of our shared memory a few weeks earlier. At the time of the benediction of our marriage, August 18, 1944, the descending sun's rays flowed through the stained glass windows of Bethel Evangelical Church and shined on us with a sign that God was blessing us as the pastor pronounced the benediction.

None of us knew what the future held. Our son Charles and daughter Lynn had been with us for the end of their mother's life. Peter and his wife Becky joined us within a day or two, as did Chuck's wife Linda, Marian's brother Roger and sister-in-law Sara, my sister Carol, who introduced us, nieces and nephews, and a multitude of friends and relatives. Roger is now the only surviving member of the Peters clan. My sister Carol and I and a few cousins are the remnants of our generation.

In the timeless plan of God, humanity is quite similar to the waves of the ocean, with each generation following the next, and in many respects, so seldom learning from the experiences of previous generations.

I think it was Shakespeare who said, "The bad that men do lives after them. The good is often interred with their bones." Certainly, Marian was human and predominantly good, which will forever be remembered.

A Chinese philosopher, Hu Shih, whose writings I admired in my youth, described immortality as something like the waves in a quiet pond produced by a stone thrown into it. The influence of a person on the lives of those around him or her will, to a lesser extent, be reflected on the lives touched by the waves of his predecessors.

While I fully expect to be reunited with Marian in the course of time in that House of Many Mansions, I am sure she will live on in the lives of those privileged to know her in this life.

1

"What Would Christ Have Me Do?"

On May 11, 1932, I quit high school with six weeks of my junior year of high school remaining in order to support the family and run our farm when my father fell down a chute of the silo, severely injuring his back. His physical injury was compounded by deep depression.

That same year, Dr. E. M. Keller, an osteopathic physician, started caring for my crippled father. He was a dedicated Methodist who was also a lay preacher. He became my close friend and introduced me to the need for social action in Christian life — not then a feature of the Lutheran Church I knew.

Dr. Keller taught me principles and techniques of osteopathy which I could use on my family members under his direction. But our sharing of books and philosophical discussions during this period led me to a closer relationship with Jesus Christ, not only as a Savior but as a friend and role model. "Why calleth me Friend and not do the things I say?"

By 1937, my father's health had improved enough that I could, at the age of twenty-one, return to high school. War clouds were already forming; newspapers and *Time* magazine accounts of world development became part of our discussions.

By that time, my earlier thoughts of becoming an agriculture teacher had been replaced by the dream of becoming an osteopathic physician. However, I enrolled in pre-med at the University of Wisconsin in Madison and eventually graduated from medical school as an MD in 1947. But I continued to associate with and learn from osteopaths.

Until the mid-1960s, it was considered unethical for MDs to associate with osteopaths, but I continued through the years to learn from osteopaths to benefit my patients. As a result, currently about eighty percent of my practice is hands-on manipulation.

Midway through my freshman year of college in 1938, I was called home to learn that my father had shot himself because of his depression over not being able to support his family. My brother Harry, four years younger than I, and my mother and sisters insisted on my continuing in school.

About the time of my father's death, Bob Gollhardt, a roommate and a fellow Lutheran, convinced me to attend Bethel Lutheran Church in Madison, then a small Norwegian Lutheran church. Morrie Wee was the pastor. I became active in the church and, in common with many others, developed an admiration and love for Morrie Wee. He had the same vision as I did of the need for each individual to have a personal relationship with Jesus Christ. The church was the vehicle by which that relationship developed and was nurtured.

During that time, the present Bethel church was built, and as we were preparing to have our first worship in the new church,

Morris wished to test the acoustical system. He asked me to go to the pulpit and read John 3:16 as he evaluated the sound in different parts of the church. What an awesome experience that was!

The reason I was at the church that day was for a counseling session with Morrie, one of many, as I struggled with the moral dilemma of selective service and my local draft board.

By the time of registration for the draft in 1939, I had, for two or three years, independently arrived at the decision that participation in war as a combatant was wrong for me. While I had never met a conscientious objector, I was aware that the Quakers, Mennonites and Church of the Brethren had a pacifist heritage. Some Methodists, of whom Dr. Keller was one, also shared their views. Morrie Wee helped me arrive at the decision that this was what Christ would have me do.

Although I knew that medical students were to be deferred, I indicated at registration for the draft in 1939 that if war came, I would be unable to accept military service. If any member of my medical school class were drafted for military service, I would choose to work, without recompense, for humanitarian organizations such as the American Red Cross, Salvation Army or American Friends Service Committee as long as other men in my class were required to serve in the armed services.

Classification as l-AO duly arrived. The local board, some of whom were members of my home church, tried to convince me to change my mind; one of those members was a cousin of my mother. He let her know that if I withdrew my statement of belief, they would never draft me, even after I graduated from medical school. As the only person in Dodge County registered as a CO, the draft board apparently thought I was an embarrassment to them. Needless to say, family and friends thought I was crazy.

During 1940 and early 1941, I not only had correspondence with the local board but with the Selective Service officers in

Madison and Washington, D.C., culminating in an appeal to President Roosevelt to allow me to remain in medical school as a conscientious objector. After the final appeal was denied in the summer of 1941, I answered my country's call in August 1941. I was assigned to "work of national importance" at the Merom, Indiana, CPS 14, run by the American Friend's Service Committee.

At the induction center in Milwaukee, I met other conscientious objectors for the first time, Stu Olbrech, a Congregationalist from Madison, and Wesley Schmidt from Sheboygan. They shared the train ride to Terre Haute and a station wagon ride to Merom, Indiana.

Before I left Madison, Dr. Middleton, dean of the medical school, called me to his office. He said he didn't understand my position, but admired my intestinal fortitude for sticking to it. He also said that while he probably wouldn't be around when it was possible for me to return to medical school, there would be a written request to his successor to reinstate me without prejudice any time I would be free to return to medical school.

Dr. Middleton himself soon became Chief Medical Officer in the European theater of World War II.

That letter was subsequently honored by Acting Dean Dr. Meek. I was re-admitted at 7:30 a.m., January 1, 1945, after many adventures, tensions and emotional turmoil.

Men assigned to alternative service were given no recompense by the government. Members of the Peace Churches supported the camps and conscientious objectors unable to pay their own way. I was one of those unable to contribute to my support and I am grateful to those who contributed beyond their means to enable those of us of like minds to live according to our convictions.

The camp at Merom CPS 14 run by the American Friend's Service Committee was under the direction of Claude Shotts and his wife Mary. He had been executive director of the Evanston, Illinois, YMCA and answered the call of conscience to volunteer his services.

While the work of the camp was to be soil conservation and I had been a farmer, it turned out I never did any farm work while at Merom. I had worked at various jobs to make my way at the university, and it was learned I had worked in restaurants in Madison. Assignment to the clean-up crew at the camp kitchen was followed by assignment to the cooking staff and finally to head cook. (I am now back to clean-up crew at home in 1992!)

The time at Merom was one of the most blessed experiences of my life. Rubbing shoulders and sharing experiences with men from seventeen different denominations, learning to experience the presence of God in the quiet Quaker worship each morning, with no liturgy but with each of us contributing to the meeting as the Spirit moved him, was a unique experience which I fondly remember. Often a meaningful message developed during these gatherings.

Informally, I became sort of a liaison between campers and administration. Some of the people in the community of Merom were supportive of the campers. Others didn't like it that a camp of "yellow bellies" was in their midst. They showed their resentment by crossing the street to avoid any contact and contamination.

One of our strongest supporters was a Methodist minister, Casey Jones, who had a church in the village as well as two smaller churches in the country. He accepted offers of help from some of the campers and frequently some of us substituted for him when he was on vacation. His people willingly listened to our amateur sermons and invited us to their homes for dinner.

My enduring recollection of Pearl Harbor is listening to the chilling news on the radio while preparing a sermon on the third floor of the Holt Institute overlooking the Wabash River.

During those months before the United States entered the war, I started writing to some of the seventeen Lutheran conscientious objectors scattered throughout the United States. Another correspondent was O. G. Malmine, editor of the Lutheran Herald. Later, when I shared with him, as well as Morrie Wee, that I felt called to the ministry, they arranged for me to meet the administrator of the Lutheran Theological Seminary, Dr. Gullickson. He indicated the board would not consider a CO as a candidate for the duration of the war, but might reconsider after the war was over.

Later, in 1953, after having practiced medicine in Jackson for four years following graduation from medical school and a year's internship at Milwaukee Hospital, run by Lutheran Sisters, I conferred with Morrie Wee about the possibility of again applying to the seminary. Since by that time I was already working with alcoholics and others in need, he said, "Jim, I think you can do more for Jesus Christ as a lay person than as an ordained member of the church."

One other recollection of my visits with Morrie during the time I was at Merom was a noonday lunch with him during a trip to Madison. He asked my opinion of the difference between the Norwegian Lutheran Church and my home church.

In my home church, I told him, I learned to know *about* Jesus Christ. At Bethel I came *to know Him* as a personal Friend as well as Savior.

During that same visit, we postulated about the possibility of a merger of the Lutheran Church for the common good and increased support for the work of God. Neither of us thought it likely in our lifetime, but by 1960, one merger was accomplished. Less than thirty years later, further mergers occurred. Whether or not these mergers will accomplish the goals we visualized is in God's hands.

Occasionally, Morrie had me go back to Bethel to tell the young people about my experiences as a CO at Merom as well as working with people from other denominations.

The one common denominator among us at Merom appeared to be that, except for the men from the Peace Churches, who had been brought up to think of pacifism as a way of life, most of us were there because our individual experiences walking with God led us to the conviction that, for us, participation as a combatant in war was wrong. Many of us, probably the vast majority, felt our country's participation in war was wrong. We were a tiny minority as the world's tensions brought us to Pearl Harbor. None of us were in a position to do as some people of that time did, voicing their opinion by withholding the taxes that supported the war effort.

The Lutheran Church seemed almost schizophrenic in its teaching that submission to the authority of the state superseded the necessity for each individual to walk with God as He directed. Kahlil Gibran expressed it well in his book, *The Prophet*: "For as each of us is alone in the knowledge of God, so is each of us alone in his knowledge of God and in his understanding of the earth."

Dramatic changes in all areas of life became apparent with the entry of the United States in active conflict. How did we reconcile our relative safety at a camp for conscientious objectors with the life-threatening events our drafted friends, now in active service, were experiencing? Were we indeed "yellow bellies" thinking only of our own safety?

These questions influenced the development of alternative service in such things as becoming human guinea pigs in medical experiments; fighting forest fires, which claimed many lives; and working in state mental institutions.

As each opportunity presented, volunteers at our camp and other CO camps exceeded the needs. Consequently, in the early spring of 1942, I was accepted to fill a call to serve at Cleveland State Hospital working with mental patients and the patients in the hospital's tuberculosis ward. I can't remember how many of us went from Merom Public Service Camp, probably five or six including Ray Hansen and Dusty Rhodes, as I recall. The COs replaced hospital workers leaving for war or higher paying industrial jobs.

It soon became apparent to me that the Catholic Chaplain, Father Murphy, and outside ministers visiting patients at the hospital had a greater influence on the well-being of the patients than the five psychiatrists on staff.

It was also apparent that "man's inhumanity to man" was present in the institution. Patient abuse, lack of compassion and discrepancies between what was actually served the patients and the dietitian's menu, was noted by the COs serving in various capacities in the different departments.

After several months of collecting data, we went to the Cleveland newspapers, resulting in an exposé of the hospital, which eventually resulted in correction of attitude and care of the mentally ill throughout the country.

My assignment as the one and only lab technician in a 2,800-bed patient facility enabled me to get on all of the wards. (God had seen fit to enable me to complete a five-credit course in physiological chemistry in summer school just before my induction to prepare me for this assignment.) Later when I was able to return to medical school, it meant I had a lesser work schedule enabling me to get used to studying again. Even so, both a *Webster's Dictionary* and a *Stedman's Medical Dictionary* were constantly at my side for months after returning to school.

In the summer of 1942, I arrived at the decision that I could become a member of the armed services as a non-combatant with the reservation that I was prepared to accept the consequences of disobeying two orders: I would not take a human life, and I would not treat wounded enemy differently than our own.

To this day, I'm not sure whether it was a romantic interest and engagement to a red-haired nurse who wanted me in service, or my rationalization that with so many of my friends in danger and dying I was honor bound to support them, which led me to compromise my principles.

My reclassification led me to Great Lakes Naval Station outside Chicago. There, the psychiatrists were interested in what had happened in Cleveland, as well as what had happened for me to change my mind and become 1-A0.

They wanted to know if I still had the same convictions of right and wrong. If in the Navy, did I expect to express my opinions to others? I admitted I probably would.

The resulting big "U" on my chest, unfit for military service, brought about a confrontation with the station's Lutheran chaplain. He listened to my story and said, "Albrecht, you go back to Madison and tell Morris Wee I am ashamed a man with your views would be a member of the Norwegian Lutheran Church." He apologized when I asked him if he was speaking as a representative of God or of the U. S. Navy. A further conference resulted in his admission that it was unfortunate that others didn't share my views.

At any rate, my red-haired nurse soon sent me a Dear John letter when she learned I was classified unfit for military service. She did keep the ring which I had bought with the proceeds of the sale of my typewriter.

At that time, people rejected by one branch of service were sent back to their local boards for reclassification. My board indicated that since I had been a farmer before medical school, I should have no objection to being a farmer again. They would not consider allowing me to return to medical school. I was assigned to the war manpower pool and became a hired man for a neighboring farmer.

Within a few months, my brother Harry, who was running the home farm as well as three other farms, entered the Navy, ultimately being on the ship where the Pacific peace treaty was signed. I returned home to help his hired men and friends run his four farms until late October or early November 1944.

One day while shopping at a grocery store in Beaver Dam, a small news article caught my eye. It was on the front page of the *Chicago Tribune* on the news rack. It said that President Roosevelt had decreed that local boards no longer could direct men in my classification.

When the secretary of the local board confirmed that the board no longer had jurisdiction over me, I contacted Dr. Meek, acting dean of the medical school. He affirmed that Dr. Middleton had indeed directed I be re-admitted without prejudice, and that if I were in class by January 1, 1945, at 7:30 a.m., I would be reinstated.

I had married on August 18, 1944, and my mother planned on remarrying in January 1945. My re-entry into medical school meant a lot of hurried readjustments in many lives. In retrospect, it is almost impossible to believe; it was possible only with the help of God.

In addition to farm chores, that fall I took a job delivering coal for Starkweather Lumber Company in Beaver Dam in order to save money for tuition due in January. My wife, who was teaching in Beaver Dam, was invited by my grandmother to stay with her in town until the end of the school year.

After her marriage in January, my mother moved to town and the farm was rented until Harry returned from service.

Further tension developed as I learned my routine skin test for medical school was positive and I had a tuberculous lesion in my right lung due to working with patients in the tuberculosis ward at the Cleveland State Hospital. Fortunately, I was allowed to remain in medical school under close observation. I had no symptoms and gastric tests remained normal.

Emotional stress produced physical symptoms of pain in my right upper chest repeatedly over the next three or four years. They appeared two or three days before the next scheduled chest x-ray, and disappeared within an hour or two of the radiologist telling me "no change," or "it seems a little smaller." This syndrome has made it easy for me to empathize with my patients, as we consider their complaints, in the context of the interrelationship of body, mind and spirit.

Despite the humiliation my stance in World War II brought on my family and myself, I believe I would have had the same views and reactions to military service in subsequent conflicts our country became involved in.

None of the conflicts accomplished their stated goals. All resulted in deaths and impoverishment of the adversaries out of all proportion to hoped-for gain. No country in history has really won a war. Humanity has lost them all!

It is my belief that each of us must, in all areas of our individual lives, honestly ask ourselves, "What would Christ have me do?" and then ask God to have the Holy Spirit give us the knowledge and strength to accomplish His purpose in our lives.

My time as a conscientious objector during World War II was only a brief interval in a lifetime of six years more than the proverbial three score and ten. I have come to realize that God, as a Master Potter, shapes and conforms our lives to His purpose by the applications of pressures we perceive of as experiences. "He is the potter, I am the clay."

CHAPTER

2

"Life Experiences"

ociety has seldom, if ever, experienced as many changes in any century as we have experienced since my birth, February 6, 1916. We have moved from largely an agricultural society to a way of life entirely different from those earlier years. The extended family, which had been so much a part of my boyhood recollections, is virtually unheard of today.

During the time I was growing up, people really meant it when they vowed, "Until death do us part." Broken homes and divorce were the exception rather than the rule. Though there may have been some illegal abortions, there was nothing like abortion on demand.

At the completion of my State Medical Board examination in June 1948, the medical examiner addressed those of us taking the exam with a word of warning. He called to our attention that we had invested a good deal of time and money, arriving at the point where we could take the exam to practice medicine. He stated that all of this would be wasted if we were ever found guilty of performing an abortion. In Wisconsin, no doctor would get his license back if he were found guilty of that one sin.

Two or three years later, at 11:30 p.m., a young woman came to my combined home-office. She had gotten off a northbound train and walked the block to my office. Because she was in a state of shock, I called upstairs to my wife Marian to come down and help me. I soon found the woman had undergone an incomplete abortion in another town.

While I was getting intravenous fluids started, Marian called Dr. Hofmeister, one of the obstetrician-gynecologists in Milwaukee I called on many times for help. Marian explained the situation to him.

The fluids and vasopressor and the oxytoxic I had started brought the woman's blood pressure out of the danger level. Dr. Hofmeister described how I should get her in stirrups and, using a sterile speculum, inspect the vagina. A sterile ring forceps should be handy, he said, in case I found, as he suspected, a fetus or a partial fetus or the placenta in the cervical os.

Marian held the phone to my ear and the mouthpiece to my mouth when I wanted to speak. Dr. Hofmeister gave me the directions as to how to remove the products of conception, to use sterile gauze to swab out the interior of the uterus, simultaneously adding Ergotrate to the intravenous solution already running.

The bleeding stopped and I was able to pack the vagina as he instructed. The patient was responsive and no longer needed the oxygen I had started prior to calling Dr.

Hofmeister. Despite the fact that the bleeding had stopped, the patient was in no condition to be allowed to go home. There was too much danger of infection. I loaded her onto the stretcher I carried in my station wagon.

We got the patient to the hospital. She required no further treatment except for antibiotics, and within a few days she was ready to go home.

The doctor who started the job lost his license and ended up selling fly traps. Nowadays, interrupting pregnancies is a well-paid specialty! Disregard for the sanctity of marriage and human life are responsible for a great many of the problems our society is experiencing today.

My grandmother Albrecht's mother, *Grossmutter* Butterbrodt we called her in German, lived in one section of the home she shared for many years with her youngest son, Arthur, his wife and family. I recall visiting her from time to time and enjoying buttered toast with a mixture of sugar and cinnamon on almost every visit. She died at age ninety-seven when I was a teenager.

Grandma and Grandpa Albrecht's home was about three-quarters of a mile away from our home farm across the fields — and a mile away by the road. *Grossmutter* Butterbrodt and Uncle Art lived about three-quarters of a mile to the east. Between these two farms was one run by a cousin of my father, August Butterbrodt and his wife Leona. Their two boys, Lawrence and Louie, were a little younger than I, but we shared many evenings of baseball after chores as we got older. Their sister Helen and younger brother Robert tagged along. Later, when I returned to work on Harry's farm in 1944, Bob was my right-hand man.

Another brother of Grandma Albrecht, Herb Butterbrodt, had a farm north of Uncle Art. In addition to farming, he was a skilled carpenter. We engaged him to remodel a bedroom in our farmhouse when Marian and I married in

1944. Herb Butterbrodt had a son, Dallas, who was a pharmacist. Another uncle of my father, Fred Butterbrodt, was already living in Beaver Dam, having turned his farm over to his son, Erwin. That farm was about three miles east of our home farm.

Those farmers, together with Otto Dinkel, our next door neighbor to the south, shared work with each other — threshing, silo filling and shredding — going from one farm to the other during the harvest seasons. The women on each farm prepared food for all the workers.

Grandma Albrecht had three sisters, the oldest of whom was married to the only other professional man in the family — Uncle Doc. Dr. Roland Schoen was his actual name. He was a family practitioner in Beaver Dam.

Grandma Albrecht's two maiden sisters and their brother Frank owned the Butterbrodt Book Store in Beaver Dam, which I visited frequently — almost every Saturday night — while growing up.

Another brother of my grandmother, Ernst Butterbrodt, lived several miles away. As I recall, he was older than the rest and had a son, Roland, who was about my father's age. He owned the threshing machine our local group of farmers used.

Grandpa Herman E. Albrecht, was a gentle, reserved man, content to let Grandmother Augusta run the household. Many times in the late spring and summer when the wind was from the southwest, he would have Grandma "ring me up" (on the hand-cranked party line phone) to see if I wanted to go fishing. Needless to say, I never said no, and proceeded to dig angle worms while waiting for him to travel the mile down the road with the horse and milk buggy.

We would then drive five or six miles to a friend who had a farm close to Beaver Dam Lake, put our horse in the barn, and walk one-half to three-quarters of a mile to the lake. For several hours we would fish for bullheads, then trudge back, hitch our horse up and get home before dark. As I got older, Grandpa Albrecht would take me to his house and we would skin bullheads for several hours by the light of kerosene lanterns.

Grandma and Grandpa Albrecht had five children. My father, Herbert E. Albrecht was born in 1888. Sisters Alma and Veronica, both of whom had normal-school educations, were country school teachers prior to their marriages.

Waldemar E. Albrecht, my uncle and godfather, shared the home farm with Grandma and Grandpa. He had been crippled with polio as a boy and had an unhappy love affair which left him a permanent bachelor and, ultimately, a problem with alcohol. Dealing with Uncle Walde's problem led me to become involved in the treatment of alcoholism in the 1950s and '60s as a part of my family practice.

My uncle Jack — Gerald was his given name — the youngest of the Albrecht children, was a salesman who first lived in Mayville, about twenty miles northeast of Beaver Dam, then in Prairie du Sac in south-central Wisconsin. After Uncle Walde died of a hemorrhage of varicose veins in his esophagus, a secondary condition brought on by his alcoholism, Uncle Jack and his wife Dorothy took care of Grandma Albrecht during her last few years of life until she died at the age of ninety-six.

Years earlier, Aunt Dorothy was instrumental in helping me get started at the University of Wisconsin when she arranged for me to be the houseboy for her mother, Mrs. Barton. Bob Gollhardt, Harold Akin and I shared the three small rooms on the top floor of Barton House. In return for taking care of the furnace and janitorial work, my room was free; and with the family connection, I also shared the kitchen, so I had some cooked meals.

31

The following year, Barton House became a women's rooming house. Mrs. Barton arranged for me to work for her sister, Mrs. Doll Howard, at a larger women's rooming house, Howard Lodge, half a block away across Mills Street. I did the janitorial work at Howard Lodge. Mrs. Barton and I continued to share meals in return for my doing janitorial work at Barton Lodge.

My mother's parents, John and Phoebe Keil, were somewhat different in that Grandpa Keil was the master of his household. He was a relatively well-to-do man with a philosophy that a happy man was a rich man. His first wife, by whom he had a daughter, my Aunt Ella, died during a second childbirth. I am not certain when he married grandma, but she brought Ella up as one of her own and subsequently had five children of her own, John, Verna, Cora (my mother), Florence and Marvin.

John married Nina Kellom, sister of Uncle Roy Kellom, husband of Aunt Alma Kellom. Verna and Florence were married to very successful farmers. Uncle Art Heuer, husband of Aunt Florence, taught me to chew tobacco at about the age of twelve while I helped him pick potatoes for fifty cents a day and room and board.

Verna's husband, Uncle Will Grebe, was the personification of the work ethic. He continued to work while battling a nasty cancer of the jaw and throat.

My mother's youngest brother, Marvin Keil, was a man of short stature. He was the only one of all my uncles and aunts to graduate from a university. Uncle Marvin was proud to be an alumnus of Lawrence University, a small, private college in Appleton, Wis. He became a successful businessman and executive, first with Central Wisconsin Canneries and then for Green Giant. It was amusing to think of my short uncle Marvin attending functions throughout the United States and recruiting missions to

Jamaica and other Caribbean Islands as the representative of the Jolly Green Giant. He certainly was jolly.

Aunt Ella married Fred Miller. Uncle Fred owned several farms, but they lived in Beaver Dam all the time I knew them. Frequently, they visited us on Sunday and we enjoyed fried potatoes and pork sausage for supper.

They had a son, Erwin. When I was about seven or eight, I was much impressed that Erwin had his own car and attended the University of Wisconsin School of Engineering. Later, he worked in the steel mills in Gary, Indiana and married Florence Mayberry. She was the sister of a featherweight boxing champion. Erwin and Florence had two sons, Fred and Bill. I remember as a youth carrying them "horseback" on my shoulders when they visited our farm.

Years later, Erwin came back to Beaver Dam to run a farm and a filling station. His son, Fred, is now retired from operating a filling station. While a second cousin, he joined the rest of the surviving Keil grandchildren at a recent reunion when Florence returned for a visit. Erwin died about fifty years ago. Florence now lives in Florida.

My mother, Cora Anna Lena Keil, born March 12, 1892, was the middle and more sturdy of the Keil daughters. As a girl, she helped with milking, washing milk cans, and other farm chores.

When she married my father in 1915, he told her she would not be permitted to do the chores or milk cows again. Little did either of them foresee the trials and tribulations that were to be their lot in life. These are a part of the fabric of my life and a part of my story. All of that generation are now deceased.

My sister Marjorie, two years younger than I, died three years ago of complications from an old bout of rheumatic heart disease. My brother Harry, four years younger than I, died after a farm construction accident in 1969. My youngest sister Carol and I are the survivors of our family.

Glen Kellom, Helen Kellom and Lois Bedtker are the remaining cousins, children of Uncle Roy and Aunt Alma.

Edward, the oldest son of the Kelloms, was one of my closest friends during my childhood and youth. He died several years ago. A sturdy man, he drove himself to the hospital when he experienced chest pain while at home with his invalid wife Ethel. He died on admission to the hospital. Ethel died a few years later.

Audrey and Joyce, children of Uncle Jack and Aunt Dorothy, survive, but haven't been seen for several years.

Cousins on my mother's side have kept in closer contact. Warren Grebe lives in Waupun to the north. Dorothy Grebe Madland lives in Bayside, a suburb of Milwaukee.

Aunt Florence and Uncle Art Heuer had a daughter, Betty, who married Russell Mauer, another successful farmer. Uncle Marvin Keil had one boy, John, by his first wife, Frances Beyer Keil, who died of cancer of the ovary; and a second son, Ward, with his second wife, Era Henderson Keil, who died in 1992. She was my last surviving aunt.

In retrospect, Aunt Frances had a profound influence on my life, even though I hadn't realized it until relatively recently. The family all felt very bad about her ovarian cancer and imminent death, leaving a son only a few months old. After catechism, "church school," I would often walk the one-half block or so to their house to visit her.

At that time, she was confined to an upstairs bedroom. I would climb to the landing on the stairway and stand there trying to control my emotions before continuing. Prior to her illness, she had placed two plaques on the wall of the landing. One was called "Edith Warton's Code." It read:

"To be honest, brave, frank, generous and compassionate. To reach forward for the fullest enjoyment of life compatible with the rights of others. To think before acting, to act without hesitation, and in every situation to retain a perspective and to behave urbanely."

I am not certain, but I think the person who wrote the words of wisdom on the second plaque was James Allen. His words went something like this:

"As you think you travel. As you love you attract. You are today where your thoughts have brought you. You will be tomorrow where your thoughts have taken you. You cannot escape the results of your thoughts. You will become as great as your noblest aspiration. You become as small as your basic desire."

Would that I had been able to follow these words of wisdom all the years of my life.

3

"Recollections of Childhood, 1916 — 1929"

Marian, my wife of forty-eight years, as an amateur psychoanalyst, postulated that my obstreperous nature, my often times negative attitude, and my need to be heard at any meeting are due to unremembered psychic trauma. She may be right.

My sister Marge arrived at our farm home when I was but twenty-two months old. Our farm house had a little bedroom adjacent to our parent's bedroom. I don't personally remember, but do recall later family discussions describing my reaction at being displaced from that small downstairs bedroom to one immediately above it upstairs. My vociferous crying all night disturbed both my parents. But my father prevailed in demonstrating "tough love," and I apparently learned the lesson that crying doesn't pay.

The farm house I grew up in now exists only in memory. It was demolished to make room for a more modern home during the time it was owned by my brother Harry.

The cornerstone of the "new" portion of our original farm house, dated 1888, was given to me by my sister-in-law Betty, when she moved from the farm several years ago.

The older portion of the house had been built before 1888 and became the kitchen wing of the house when the addition was built. The two wings of the house had been so skillfully joined it was hard to tell they had not been constructed together. Both sections were built of similar brick and even the basement walls failed to show where they joined.

The basement room on the east had a large cistern that provided a source of soft water, initially brought to the kitchen level by a hand pump. A potato bin and storage area occupied the remaining space in the room under the kitchen. Thick stone walls covered with plaster separated this room from the furnace room, which occupied the space under the living room. The U-shaped extension under the bay window of the living room served as a coal bin. The combination coal and wood furnace was placed in such a way that the heat rose through the floor immediately above it in an area between the door to my parent's bedroom and the door leading to the upstairs. The nickel-plated grate, about four feet in diameter, had the word "Homer" on it. Many times on cold winter mornings, after father had stoked the furnace, we children stood around "Homer" as we dressed.

The third room in the basement was an irregularly shaped "L" serving as a storage area for vegetables, canned meat and lard, as well as eggs. A stairway to the outside opened onto a concrete pad in the "L" formed by the two wings of the home. In the middle of this pad was a well with a windmill directly above it.

North of the windmill was an attached frame building. The

room closest to the house served as a laundry room for my mother. Just beyond that was a woodshed with a communicating door.

Between the building housing the laundry and the corner of the house was an arched walkway leading west, with a stone path to a grove of pine trees. Here rested a two-seater outhouse with its Sears Roebuck or Montgomery Ward catalogs. These served both as reading material and toilet paper. This outhouse was still serving its purpose when, as a boy of ten, I was asked to empty the "slop jar" containing the placenta of my newborn sister Carol. (All four of us children were born at home, delivered by Uncle Doc Schoen.)

The floor plan of our house was simple. One entered the kitchen from the north, two steps above the level of the concrete pad across from the laundry building. There were two small rooms at the east end of the kitchen wing; the bathroom and the pantry. In addition to the sink, tub, and toilet, the bathroom had clothing hooks, and it also accommodated a narrow stairway, rising over the tub, to a hall leading to the "hired man's room." Adjacent to this hall was also a storage tank which, until 1937, supplied running water to the bathrooms and kitchen by gravity, after having been pumped by the windmill to the second floor. In 1937, when electricity came to our farm, the gravity system became obsolete. The hand pump providing soft water from the cistern was also replaced with an electric pump.

A door on the south side of the kitchen opened onto a small open porch which was used only during the summer months.

One of my fondest memories was of our combination coal and wood burning stove with a reservoir to provide hot water and an oven for baking. It also provided additional heat in cold weather when the oven door was left open. Thick stove lid covers provided cooking area surfaces as well as for heating flat irons for ironing. My olfactory sense still savors the memory of the meals cooked so long ago and the yeasty fragrance of baking bread and rolls. The stove's pipe vent angled its way to the brick chimney and was cleaned frequently to avoid chimney fires.

A mantel clock was on a shelf on the west wall of the kitchen. On one side of it was a door to the living room; on the other side, an arch opened onto a small hall with three doors, one to the basement stairs, the one on the left to the living room and the one on the right to the small bedroom from which I had been evicted as a toddler.

The hired man's room above the kitchen had another door opening to the landing of the front stairway, coming up from the living room. Three steps up from the landing was the upstairs hall with a railing around the stairwell. There were three bedrooms, the small one where I spent the night crying, a large one which I later shared with my brother Harry and eventually with my wife Marian, and one slightly larger above the living room shared by my two sisters, Marjorie and Carol.

Just to the west of the house were two large maple trees, apparently the reason for the name "Maple Hill Farm."

A dirt road, one-half mile in length, led west to State Highway 151. If you turned to the left at State Highway 151, you traveled to Beaver Dam, two and one-half miles to the south. A turn to the right would take you to Waupun, about ten miles north. One-half mile south on State Highway 151 was Jefferson School District No. 2, a red brick structure where, at the age of six, I started my school career. Another dirt road from our driveway proceeded south and connected with County Highway A.

Those dirt roads became rutted in the spring and fall. Both the wagons and buggies, as well as the Model T and Model A Fords had enough clearance. Getting stuck in either mud or snow was less common than would be experienced by our more modern cars of today.

Later on, these roads became gravel and are now blacktopped.

As you proceeded west from our driveway, there were seven stately evergreen trees, on the right, with a fence constructed from the stones laboriously "harvested" each spring from the farm fields. On the left of the road was a stone fence on our neighbor Otto Dinkel's farm. At that point, his land was very low. Almost always in the spring and fall, it was covered with water, which attracted ducks and geese.

We had two low lying areas on our farm, one a little northwest of Dinkel's pond. This apparently didn't have the same clay structure because the water never stood there more than a few days. However, a pasture north of the farm buildings and home had a larger pond area with blue clay under the soil. This pond would keep water for months, and invariably was the stopping place for ducks and geese on their spring and fall migrations. It also was the site to which our cows came to drink and cool off. Later in my boyhood this pond was the site where Marge, Harry and I went one memorable occasion for an unauthorized "swim." Spankings resulted from both Father and Mother. This was in the era when parents were expected to discipline their children without fear of being accused of abuse.

In my opinion, "sparing the rod and spoiling the child" is responsible for many of today's social problems. Without respect for parental authority, our young people are conditioned to show a lack of respect for teachers and all authority figures to the detriment of themselves, as well as of society.

The two "forties" (fields) to the east of the farmstead also had some stone fences, a woven-wire fenced area where animals were to be kept from time to time, and some barbed wire fencing.

During my early boyhood and youth, herbicides had not been thought of. The fence rows had many blackberry bushes, which yielded good fruit. As we children got old enough, we picked berries to be made into jelly and jars of canned berries to be stored on the shelves in our basement for winter use.

Wild roses and other perennial flowers shared the fence row with the wild raspberries. In some places, maple and box elder trees had gained a foothold. Of course, the weeds, Canada thistles and burdocks had to be cut every year to prevent them from seeding and propagating in the adjacent fields.

At the junction of our farm and Uncle Walde's was a gate leading from our back forty to his back forty. Later in my boyhood, this was the path I frequently took when hiking over to visit Grandma and Grandpa, Uncle Walde and Aunt Ronnie, when she was not teaching school. It also provided a convenient path for driving farm implements from one farm to the other.

So much for the geography of my memories of long ago.

Tangible mementos of the past include the old library table at which I am now sitting and once part of the furnishings in the little bedroom of my old home. Frequently during the late '20s and early '30s, I sat at this table balancing my books for various 4-H projects. The table was given to me by my mother ten or fifteen years ago and is one of my prized possessions.

At this table, in 1933, my crippled father had me type an article he was never able to sell, based on his alarm at the ever increasing federal debt. As I recall, at the time of my father's concern, the national debt was about $15.5 billion! His concern was well-founded. By 1940, two years after his death, it had escalated to $42.9 billion. Ten years later it was at $257.3 billion. In 1992 it was said that the current national debt was up to four trillion dollars. Without a drastic change of direction and reduction of the current, almost impossible to imagine, debt, this country as we have known it cannot long survive.

Economists must feel almost as apprehensive as a physician feels when a patient comes in with a long neglected carcinoma, which has metastasized to all parts of the body!

Another heirloom in my possession is a highchair which was used in turn by me, Marge, Harry and Carol, and then by nine grandchildren and eight great-grandchildren as they visited my mother until her death. This old, often painted (currently white) highchair sits in the corner of our dining room with a rag doll, Ruby Sue, the current occupant. The tray, fastened with an unusual lock, swivels outward and probably will never again be used for its intended purpose. It currently serves as a resting place for things we have to remember to take downstairs. Ultimately, it probably will be given to the Washington County Historical Society.

Each time I go into our garage, I see on a shelf the white slop jar in which I carried my sister Carol's placenta to the outhouse a little over sixty-five years ago. It is a functional pail for other purposes now.

A fourth heirloom is an oval etched glass design of a girl, a horse, and a dog. This etched glass was originally the window in the south door of the living room of my Grandpa and Grandma Albrecht's home, and the object of my admiration as a youth on my frequent visits.

When that house was being remodeled by a new owner in 1975, we stopped and spoke to the priest who was converting it to a home for disadvantaged boys. The door, with its window, had already been removed and stored in the old laundry. He saw that it meant a great deal to our family. He gave it to us, and graciously accepted a donation for his project. We had the old door taken apart and the etched glass mounted in our dining room door leading to the deck. Each time I eat a meal at home I think of the Albrecht family of long ago.

One additional memento of the past is an old wood box that I commissioned Grandfather Albrecht to make as a present for my mother when I was about five or six years old. He made it out of scraps of lumber. While he didn't want to charge me for it, he did accept two and a half dollars, which I had saved from my weekly allowance of twenty-five cents. I had saved the money over a few months by foregoing the fifteen cent ice cream sundaes I usually had as a feature of our Friday night shopping in downtown Beaver Dam. Mother gave the wood box to me about ten or fifteen years ago.

As I dictate this, with tears coming to my eyes, I reflect what wonderful things memories are. Even as I reflect, I feel sorry for the many people who dwell on bad memories. I have a few bad memories, but by and large have been richly blessed with good memories as you will see as we progress through the story of my life.

4

"More Recollections of Childhood"

World War I was well underway at the time of my birth. I am sure I don't truly recall the Armistice. What I think I remember may be the joy and celebration on November 11, 1918.

I remember the fear of the flu epidemic in 1919; my parents and grandparents discussed the untimely deaths of those who succumbed. In later years, people a few years older than I who had gone through the epidemic were thought to have that as the cause of their affliction with Parkinson's Disease.

I have no recall of President Woodrow Wilson, who served between 1913 and 1921, though I remember relatives speaking disparagingly of "that Democrat." It is still hard for me to understand how the disadvantaged Albrecht family ended up being Republicans. It is easy to understand that my more well-off maternal relatives were of that political persuasion.

I do recall seeing the headlines when President Warren G. Harding died in 1923, and my personal recollection of Calvin Coolidge (Silent Cal) is a mental picture of him fishing for trout at a northern Wisconsin resort sometime during my boyhood.

I have vivid recollections of the psychic shock from the reversal of family and national fortunes during the Great Depression. This makes it easy to remember Herbert Hoover.

I still tingle as I remember hearing on the battery-operated radio Franklin Delano Roosevelt give his inaugural address in 1933, proclaiming, "The only thing we have to fear is fear itself."

Our farm home, in common with many homes of that day, had hardwood floors and throw rugs rather than the wall-to-wall carpet of today. The kitchen was the only really warm room in the winter. Saturday night baths were accomplished in a laundry tub placed next to the stove, the oven door open to shed even more warmth on the shivering children and adults. In later years, a portable kerosene heater would warm the bathroom after we had a bathtub.

The reservoir on the stove provided a portion of the water for the weekly baths, with large kettles on top of the stove providing the rest. The younger children were bathed first and put to bed. So, being the oldest, I was always the last to bathe.

I recall lying on the wooden floor next to the stove watching my hard-working mother scurry around getting us three meals a day and, at least once a week, scrubbing the floor on her hands and knees. While she didn't have to help with the milking, as many farm women did, she was kept busy tending chickens and our large garden. Women of that era did a lot of sewing, especially mending. I recall a saying heard frequently in my boyhood, "A man works from sun to sun, but a woman's work is never done."

We children were taught at an early age, as each one came along — first me, then Marge, Harry, and ten years after me,

Carol — the need for family cohesiveness, with each of us providing love and support for the other.

The extended family relationships on both sides were warm, in spite of our being the "poor relation" financially. Thanksgiving was celebrated at Grandpa and Grandma Keil's home, and Christmas at the home of Grandma and Grandpa Albrecht. In the early days, horse and buggy or bobsled was our means of getting there, especially if roads would not permit the early cars to negotiate the rutted dirt roads or the snow.

The women on both the maternal and paternal sides of the family were excellent cooks. Each family would bring an assigned dish, with the hostess preparing the fowl and potatoes. One of my favorite desserts was Glorified Rice and, of course there were always apple, pumpkin, and cherry pies.

In the spring of 1922 my father took me in our Nash car to the one-room Jefferson School District No. 2 to introduce me to the person who would be my teacher throughout grade school, Miss Emma Elser. Several more visits that spring took away my apprehension of starting school that fall. I became acquainted with other children as isolated as we were.

Some fifty years later it was an emotional shock for me when I visited Miss Elser in a nursing home.

Later, Jefferson School was the place where there would be box socials and 4-H club meetings. It was where we learned to salute the flag every morning, where we vied for the opportunity to get water from the well, and to bring in the coal to stoke the round oak stove.

Miss Elser would arrive at the school one-half hour early so she could have the place warmed up — at least we didn't have to have our mittens on during school hours! When the weather was rainy or snowy, our outer clothing and boots were brought into the school room to dry near the stove. When dry, they were kept in the hall cloak room, but brought in again to be warmed by the stove before it was time to go home.

During the school day, it was common for children to go to the front of the room as their class was called to recite lessons. The rest of us were supposed to be studying until it was our turn to recite. All during the school year, the older children helped the younger ones with their studies.

Many children with that type of education did pretty well in life, since there was peer pressure to do one's best.

I think my almost illegible writing is partly due to having skipped seventh grade after passing an achievement test in the spring of my sixth year at school. At that time, Dodge County was experimenting with rewarding "gifted children" by speeding up their educational process. I have wondered if some of my social maladjustments and poor writing habits may have been due to missing that one grade.

Farm children at that time, or at least in our family, were taught the need to do chores to help the family survive, as well as to teach each individual the necessity of pulling his own weight. Early chores included gathering eggs, shucking sweet corn in season, pulling weeds in the garden, and a little later, washing cow udders prior to milking. Harry's and my apprenticeship included cleaning cattle alleyways, gutters, and stalls in the barn, then feeding the cows. We learned to curry the horses and feed them hay and a measure of oats. Later on, as we gained strength and stature, we hauled out the manure from the barns with a wheelbarrow.

Not until later boyhood were we entrusted with cleaning the bull's pen, and then only if the bull was secured to the wall by a ring in his nose so he wouldn't damage us when we invaded his sanctuary.

Long before the "state-of-the art" conveyor system of today, which automatically takes manure from the gutters to the barnyard pile, we had an overhead track with a manure carrier. This extended about one hundred and fifty feet east of the barn. It was supported with poles and made a U-shaped turn inside the barn, providing access to all the gutters behind the cows. This carrier could be raised or lowered by pulling on a chain attached to cog wheels so that the manual labor of lifting the manure with a fork was reduced, somewhat. We only had to lift the twenty- to thirty-pound forksful of manure three feet rather than four or five.

Cleaning the barn as well as feeding the cows was a twice-a-day chore.

At about the age of six or seven, under the supervision of Grandpa Albrecht, I was allowed to lead the horse on a rope to raise the hay fork, embedded in a layer of hay in the hay rack, to the top of the barn. A track carried it and deposited it for stacking in the hay mow.

My father and Uncle Walde shared the haying as well as other farm operations. Uncle Walde had a harpoon fork (two tines) and we had a grapple fork (four tines). Each man or boy had a specific job during haying. Operations were orderly and coordinated by "shop jargon," with one wagon being loaded in the field while another was unloaded at the barn.

This was a sweaty, dirty job for all involved, but a part of being a farmer. As I matured, I did some of the heavier jobs. During my teens, I once had a heat stroke in the hay mow.

One of my fondest recollections is my being entrusted at the age of seven to start doing farm work during the spring seeding ritual.

A pair of gray mares, Lady and Dolly, were attached to a twelve-foot drag. I learned to drive them without the drag and then, under Grandpa Albrecht's supervision, trudge along as he demonstrated how to cross the field and turn without tipping the drag over. After a few of these maneuvers, the reins were given to me to put around my back. I had already learned to say "Giddyup" and "Whoa."

For a few turns Grandpa followed me closely and then pronounced that I was ready to make a round on my own while he sat in the shade under a tree by the stone fence at the end of the field.

Under the tutelage of Grandpa Keil, who would take me with a horse and buggy out to one of his farms where he maintained a little garden, I learned to till, plant and weed a garden. Sometimes he gave me fifty cents or a dollar for a half day's work. Occasionally, I would go to Grandma Albrecht's garden where she showed me how to do things. Early in life, I helped my mother with the garden which, in the years of the Depression, became a cornerstone of our financial survival.

It wasn't until I was ten or twelve that I was entrusted to drive a two-horse team on the cultivators. Even then, I sometimes cultivated out some of the corn instead of just the weeds. Later on, there were two-row cultivators with three horses and more disastrous results if I had been up too late the night before.

Somewhat later, I learned to plow with a two-horse team and a walking plow, then with a three-horse team and a riding, "two-bottom" gang plow. It was a challenge to plow a straight furrow and later to plant a straight row of corn.

I remember the threshing crew of long ago. My father's cousin, Roland Butterbrodt, had a steam engine which required an accompanying horse-drawn water wagon and pulled a belt-driven threshing machine. At threshing time, my father, our hired man, Uncle Walde, our next door neighbor, and all the Butterbrodts who farmed within a five-mile area comprised the threshing crew. I remember the "litany" as they gathered: "Good morning Herb; Good morning Otto; Morning Augie; Morning Erv," and so on.

After the grain had been cut, tied and shocked, it was allowed to dry for two or three weeks. Threshing would not start until the dew was off the unthreshed grain so that the grain, later stored in the grainery, would not spoil or cause spontaneous fires.

The shocks were broken up with pitchforks, the sheaves thrown onto the wagon where they were stacked to a height of eight or ten feet. The wagon was then driven to either side of the platform with the conveyor belt at one end of the threshing machine. Each sheaf was pitched head first onto the platform and conveyed into the threshing machine. The straw was blown out through an adjustable metal pipe onto the straw stack wherever the farmer wanted it located. Near the middle of the machine was another six-inch pipe to which bags could be attached by hooks to receive the grain. The flow was controlled by a hand-operated baffle.

My Grandpa Albrecht was the person who supervised filling the bags. He also taught me to tie a "Miller's knot."

The bags were lined up on the ground next to the threshing machine until another two-horse team and driver arrived with a box wagon to transport the newly threshed grain to the grain bin or grainery.

The threshing process would continue from one farm to the next until the grain on all the farms was processed. The noonday meal was prepared by the women of the family where the work was being done that day. Occasionally, if rain was forecast, they would prepare a second meal so the men could work a few extra hours. However, it was a necessity that horses and wagons get back to the home farm before dark. My mother always used her best china when she served the crew at our farm.

Later in the season, the same crews gathered to fill the silos. It is interesting to note that in those early days of the Gehl Manufacturing Company in West Bend, one of the founders, Frank Gehl, actually came to our farm to demonstrate to our crew his newest silo filler.

The children were not allowed to participate in this rather dangerous job. I remember being allowed, at about age fourteen, to assist the man inside the silo as he guided the flexible pipe so that the falling chopped corn, now called silage, could be evenly distributed.

The silo's access doors at each level of silage were sealed with clay mud until the silo was filled, usually in two or three days. Then the pipes and equipment were dismantled to be hauled and reassembled at the next farm. Assembling and attachment were tricky because some silos were concrete, others stave, and their sizes varied. During these procedures corn from the field was cut by a binder and loaded onto wagons by other members of the crew.

Ideally, everything went like clockwork. But sometimes there were problems. Care had to be taken that no stones were conveyed into the silo filler and extreme caution taken that no hands or bodies were inadvertently lost.

Farming remains a hazardous occupation, though farmers of today would not recognize farms of yesteryear.

Several weeks after the silo filling operation was concluded, the remaining mature corn was cut with binders into bundles of perhaps fifteen to twenty stalks of ripe corn. These were automatically tied by the binder. The farmer and his helper would make a tepee-like shock of corn of perhaps fifteen bundles. These were allowed to dry for three to six weeks and were then ready for the tractor-driven shredder, which traveled the same route the threshing and silo-filling crews followed.

The shredder was a little different from the threshing machine in that the bundles were placed on the conveyor which pulled them into the machine. The ears were separated and husks came out the side of the machine. The stalks and leaves were chopped up and blown out a pipe at the end. These were blown into either the barn or in a stack to be used for fodder or bedding. The ears of corn were dropped into a box wagon to be hauled to a corn crib and then laboriously shoveled through the open doors, which were about shoulder height.

Corn cribs were constructed in such a way that air could

circulate to dry the corn. A few are still standing on some of the farms in our section of Wisconsin, but are seldom used in this era of large-scale farming. With modern machinery, two or three men can do as much in one day as our crew of seven farmers and their helpers could do in a couple of weeks.

Electricity didn't come to our farm until 1937. Uncle Walde, Grandma and Grandpa had it a year or two earlier. We didn't even have a battery-operated radio in 1927. In that year, I recall walking a half mile south of our home farm to the home of Art Keyser to lie on his kitchen floor and listen to the description of Lindberg's arrival in Paris.

That year, I also listened to a broadcast of the Dempsey-Tunney fight in the same farm home. I don't recall if it was the first or second fight, but it was exciting.

5

"Later
Childhood"

Farmers in Dodge County were just being introduced to scientific farming in the 1920s. The impetus was the Smith-Hughes Act passed by Congress in 1917, which gave the government the power to establish a national program of vocational education. Initially, it permitted the government to pay half the cost of the vocational agricultural program in each state. Over the years, this grant has been reduced.

By the mid-1920s Beaver Dam High School had an Ag Department supervised by Mr. L. R. Larson. Long before I entered high school in 1929, I became acquainted with him. He visited farms in our area and promoted education for the farm youth as well as encouraged farmers to use new methods to increase productivity and income.

He led the movement to make farm folk realize the need for

their children to have more than an eighth-grade education and encouraged youths to think of taking agricultural courses in high school. He urged farmers to not only improve production of their farms and herds, but to improve the productivity of their children.

Farmers were skeptical and slow to accept "school teacher" methods. But Mr. Larson gradually gained converts to improved farming practices through the local 4-H clubs, which formed a nucleus for his agricultural classes at Beaver Dam High School.

By 1929, when I entered high school, many of the more progressive farmers were already using newer methods for soil conservation, crop rotation, and to upgrade breeding stock for both dairy and meat cattle, as well as other livestock. Now, sixty years later, contour farming has become very visible throughout Wisconsin and the entire Midwest. Skilled farmers conserve their soil and create beautiful "patchwork" landscapes in the process.

4-H clubs were just being started in our area when I was ten, so I became a member of the local 4-H club and later, in 1929, entered high school as a charter member of the Future Farmers of America.

The 4-H club motto, "Make the best better," was to be achieved through the following objectives:

1. Gain knowledge, skills and qualities for a happy home life.

2. Enjoy useful work, responsibility and satisfaction in accomplishments.

3. Value research and learn scientific methods for making decisions and solving problems.

4. Know how scientific agriculture and home economics relate to the total economy.

5. Explore career opportunities and continue needed education.

6. Appreciate nature, understand conservation, and use resources wisely.

7. Foster healthful living, purposeful recreation, and constructive leisure.

8. Strengthen personal standards and philosophies.

9. Acquire traits, attitudes, and understanding to work well with others.

10. Develop leadership talents and abilities to become better citizens.

Meetings were held monthly, usually in one of the local one-room schools, or sometimes in a member's home. The 4-H club pledge was recited at each meeting:

> "I pledge my head to clearer thinking,
> My heart to greater loyalty,
> My hands to larger service and
> My health to better living
> For my club, my community, and my country."

Adult leaders provided direction and supervision, as well as encouragement for participation in group activities. Usually there were educational talks, frequent demonstrations of various projects, and always some type of game or dance, with a lunch prepared by the girls who were in home economics classes. During the meetings, we learned Roberts Rules of Order and frequently discussed our various individual projects.

My projects included gardening, raising capons and raising Duroc Jersey hogs. One year, I recall putting on a demonstration at the Dodge County Fair on caponizing (castrating) roosters. Capons were then considered a delicacy. With Mr. Larson's help, I also started a small apple orchard.

One of the most embarrassing moments of my life occurred in my third or fourth year of 4-H club membership. In an election for officers, I was nominated for president. Of course, I realized I was by far and away the logical choice, but I nominated another member.

I was greatly embarrassed when he didn't get any votes, including mine! Certainly, it was a good demonstration of the need to follow the precept, "To thine own self be true. What follows then, as night the day, thou cannot then be false to any other man."

Dr. Keller, and later my wife, postulated that my apparent high self-esteem is really overcompensation for my actual sense of inferiority in many areas.

1929 was almost a disaster for me. In the spring, Harry and I accompanied our father on a trip to buy seed barley from a farmer living a few miles from our home. As Dad and Mr. Reichert were visiting, Harry and I chased each other around the barn, climbing from one rafter to another.

As we reached the top of the barn, I was swinging from one four-by-four to the next. One broke loose and I fell thirty-five feet onto a pile of straw, carrying the four-by-four with me. At the time, the only damage seemed to be to my dignity. I did have a backache; three years later, Dr. Keller discovered that I had actually broken a vertebra in my lumbar spine. In those three years, arthritic changes had already occurred in that area of my spine, as shown by Dr. Keller's x-ray machine.

In early August of 1929, a three-horse team attached to a manure spreader ran away with the front wheel running over my head and the back wheel over my right hip. I was taken to Lutheran Hospital on the shores of Beaver Dam Lake to have the head laceration cleaned and sutured. I ended up in the hospital for four days, and then on crutches for four months.

My 4-H project that year was raising five Duroc Jersey hogs, which I had bought that spring as piglets for twenty-five dollars each from a friend of my father. The hogs had been entered in the livestock show at the Wisconsin State Fair as part of my project. I couldn't attend the fair, and my hogs were shown by my brother Harry. We did receive several blue ribbons, both at the State Fair and later at the Dodge County Fair.

For the first month or two of my freshman year in high school, I stayed with Grandma and Grandpa Keil at their home, about six blocks from the school. That way, my family didn't have to transport me the two and one-half miles every day from home.

Mr. Larson was my teacher, both in agriculture and in home room. For a few years, my goal was to become an agriculture teacher like him, and I became a charter member of the school's Future Farmers of America. Almost all of the boys in Future Farmers were sons of farmers. While we shared a common work heritage, some of us were lower on the totem pole than others financially. Despite that, there was a common sense of fellowship in seeing first hand what we were learning about in books.

Each fall there would be a trip to Madison where Future Farmers from all over the state would gather for a few days of fellowship and learning. This was held on the School of Agriculture campus at the university. I have fond memories of not only the comradeship and sense of destiny, but also of the buttermilk and ice cream. Those flavors mingle with my memories of the Babcock testing for butterfat and other, then new, farming practices.

Most of the Future Farmers also had experience in 4-H and continued, as I did, after four years of being 4-H club members to become club leaders for varying periods of time. While I didn't graduate with my original high school class of 1933, I have occasionally been invited to their reunions. I look forward to attending the sixtieth reunion this year, and hope to see many of those with whom I shared a common interest in the days of our youth.

I remained active in 4-H until the mid-1930s.

Religious instruction was accomplished in a six-week stint during the summer months preceding my freshman year at Beaver Dam High School, and continued with weekly Saturday morning sessions until confirmation. My memories of those days consist of a sense of awe at having our pastor of over twenty-five years, Reverend Gammerlien, demonstrate on the blackboard his command of Hebrew, Latin and Greek, and his insistence on our committing to memory various passages in the Lutheran Catechism. The latter was to ensure that we became word perfect in order to pass the public examination during the church service held the Sunday before our confirmation.

I am afraid most of my fellow classmates had no more personal relationship with God and Jesus Christ than I did at that point. I subsequently learned from association with members of other denominations, including Methodist, Baptist, Congregationalist, Presbyterian and Quakers, as well as other branches of the Lutheran Church, the importance of a personal relationship with Jesus Christ and the need for social involvement. This led me back to thinking of the validity of the Future Farmer's motto: "Learning to do. Doing to learn. Learning to live. Living to serve."

There were many times during the mid-1930s when I felt closer to God working in my orchard than I did going to church, where I would often fall asleep, even while standing during the liturgical service!

But during the late 1930s, I came to regard going to church on Sunday as a sort of recharging or refueling experience, thinking of myself as a car needing my battery recharged or my spiritual fuel tank refilled.

In these days of increased sexual permissiveness, controversy over how to teach the young about sex, concerns about AIDS and the resurgence of syphilis and gonorrhea, I am reminded of the five or ten minute lecture my father gave Harry and me in 1930, when an unwed neighbor girl became pregnant.

Premarital and extramarital sex were not totally unknown in previous generations, but they were not nearly as common as they have become in the last forty years. This prevalence coincides with the ever-increasing suggestiveness in movies and, in the last twenty years, permissiveness on television. The modern interpretation of the right of free speech guaranteed by our founding fathers in the Constitution must be making them turn over in their graves as they reflect on how their good intentions have been perverted by our Supreme Court.

That day in 1930, Dad called a meeting in the hog house. As he was talking, we observed the shoats and sows drinking from the trough and eating from the self-feeder. Of course, we had witnessed the sexual activity of livestock and assisted at the birth of calves and little pigs. We also had observed the castration of little boars to make them shoats, with subsequent development more conducive to good pork than had they remained boars. We were not unaware that people, in some respects, were like animals, but had not previously been taught "the facts of life" relating to humans.

Dad started out by saying, "Boys, you probably heard that our neighbor girl is going to have a baby. She doesn't have a husband. Some S.O.B. did that to her. How would you feel if somebody got one of your sister's pregnant without marrying her? Remember, every girl has a father or a brother who feels the same way about her and they probably feel as you do that you should shoot him.

"While we are on this subject, I'm telling you to keep the instrument you have between your legs in your pants, except to urinate, until you are married. I also want to let you know about a friend I knew who got a bad disease and his cock rotted off! There are two diseases, syphilis and gonorrhea, that men get when they play 'round with women. One of them makes you very sore and you have trouble urinating. The other one gets you sore a few weeks later and then in a couple of years, your brain starts deteriorating.

"Behave yourselves!"

Prohibition started in 1918 and terminated in 1932. It was an unpopular law and largely ignored. Home brew and wine were winked at and enjoyed by many. Bootleg whiskey was not unknown, and many "respectable" people made fortunes flouting the law. Gangsters were almost regarded as folk heroes. At our high school, one of the boys, fondly called "Alkie" McGreggor, took trips south in a car with hidden compartments to buy bootleg whiskey. He made enough money to be the envy of all.

Even my otherwise law-abiding father and Uncle Walde were observed to have a bottle secreted in the barn to use "as the spirit moved them."

It was not considered inappropriate at family gatherings for youngsters to be allowed to sip homemade wine and I do recall many times being asked to help mash grapes for wine and pick dandelions during the spring. I do recall the smoothness of the dandelion wine. It wasn't until later years that I learned of the dangers of getting hooked on wine and tobacco.

During the days of the flapper, smoking cigarettes became as common as the use of heroin had been twenty or thirty years earlier. Both men and women smoked. Many men chewed tobacco and successful men smoked cigars. Corncob pipes were used by the poor. Meerschaum pipes were smoked by the more well-to-do men, and briar pipes by the "Average Joe."

Kids at age twelve and thirteen started emulating their elders, making corn silk cigarettes to start, then buying a fifteen cent pack of Bull Durham tobacco and a nickel's worth of cigarette wrappers, learning to roll their own. Subsequently, they graduated to Camel and Lucky Strike cigarettes, which were, as I recall, about fifteen cents a pack.

I started smoking at the age of fifteen, interrupted it for a few years when I was interested in boxing and wrestling, and then graduated to a pipe in the mid-1930s.

I would quit for a few months from time to time, sometimes for as long as ten months at a time, only to start again. Had I not burned my pipes on May 14, 1992, I would probably be smoking as I dictate this.

People, in common with other members of the animal kingdom, are creatures of habit, and there are many substances, including alcohol and tobacco, as well as sedating and stimulating drugs, that have physical and physiologic effects likely to have deleterious effects on the lives of the users. Just this week, the *Milwaukee Journal* had an article indicating that even caffeinated coffee is habituating. While I had one earlier this morning, I am now going to have my second cup!

While 1929 was the beginning of the Great Depression, it would be another year or two before its effects struck our family. As prices went down, our income grew insufficient to meet obligations.

On May 9, 1932, I attended a happy Mother's Day dinner at the home of Uncle Art and Aunt Florence; and on May 11, my world seemed to crash around me. That day my father fell thirty-five feet from a silo. His injuries crippled him.

On that day, with six weeks left of my junior year to complete, I quit high school in order to manage the farm and support the family for the next four years. My teachers rallied to see that I got credit for my junior year. Mr. Larson taught me to drive the family car. Another teacher, Miss Rasmussen, lent me her own typewriter to practice on so I could achieve a passing grade of thirty-five words per minute. Mr. Smith, my history teacher; Miss Jax, my speech teacher; and Miss Lampert, my English teacher, gave me homework to do and saw that they were available for questioning and extra tutoring. As a consequence, when I was able to return to high school in the fall of 1936, I didn't have to repeat my junior year.

6

"The Great Depression and Change of Direction"

I don't remember how long my father remained hospitalized after his fall, but he was never again, either physically or emotionally, the same. Beside the problems of the Depression, he had to deal with his personal depression. Unable to make a living for his family, he also agonized over losing the western twenty acres of our farm because we couldn't pay the chattel mortgage. A few months later, three of our best producing cows were repossessed because we couldn't pay the six hundred dollar chattel mortgage on them.

The sense of failure and frustration was not helped by comparing the lot of his family with the families of his more successful in-laws. He did feel bad that I quit school, but we all clung to the hope that, ultimately, I would return and resume my studies.

Within a few months, finances dictated drastic measures. Our one-ton truck was put up on blocks when we couldn't replace the tires or buy gas. Then the Lawson gasoline engine which provided the energy to operate the milking machine was "put in moth balls." Even though the price of gas was only seventeen or eighteen cents a gallon, we just couldn't afford it. For a while, Harry helped me hand milk our seventeen cows. Dad was not able to do any of the physical work but was able to give us direction.

A sense of pride kept us from asking for help when, according to today's standards, we would have been very eligible.

When calves were ready to be sold for veal, at the age of four to six weeks and a weight of one hundred and twenty-five to one hundred and thirty pounds, I would take the back seat out of our Nash car, wrap the calf in canvass and, with the help of my mother, crawl into the back of the car, holding the calf in my lap and arms. My mother would drive to the stockyard and we would get three and a half or four dollars for the calf.

Every Saturday, the same car conveyed my mother and me to town where we had an egg route. Our customers got first class eggs at a few cents less than they would pay at the store and we got a few cents more than we would have gotten selling them to the store.

In season, our good-sized strawberry bed added to the family income. Mother and I would get up at four and she would go to the strawberry bed while I did the milking. After the chores were done, we would have breakfast and I would then go out and help pick the berries. We would both go to Beaver Dam and deliver them to our regular egg customers. We sometimes would butcher chickens and deliver them to our customers.

Family and friends were supportive, but we were too proud to ask for financial help. I don't recall any help being offered by my mother's relatives. Uncle Walde, and Grandma and

Grandpa Albrecht offered what help they could. Mother and Grandma worked together with the laundry at Grandma's house when we couldn't afford gas for the engine that ran our washing machine.

We shared and exchanged help with the twice-a-year butchering and making sausage from hogs raised on the farm, as well as once a year sharing a side of beef.

Prior to the advent of freezers quite a few years later, sausage and meat were usually stored in crocks covered by lard, or in glass jars stored in the cool basement of our farm house.

Milk and cream, as well as food that needed to be kept cool, were stored on a shelf in the well, constructed over the pipes about six feet below the level of the concrete pad just outside the kitchen door. Later on, this also stored homemade ice cream.

During that period, milk was picked up by a milk truck and conveyed to a Kraft milk processing plant in Beaver Dam. Uncle Walde's milk was still being conveyed to a country cheese factory about a mile from his home. During my earlier boyhood, I sometimes accompanied him in the milk buggy. But by the time of my father's accident, Uncle Walde had a half-ton truck.

Early in our marriage, Marian and I would often stop at Charlie Bachofen's local cheese factory, to buy cheese where so many years earlier I would help deliver milk.

Farmers have long since stopped using these little country cheese factories. But during an earlier era, they were scattered throughout our section of Wisconsin.

It is unlikely that without the close relationship and help of Grandma and Grandpa Albrecht we would have been able to remain self-sufficient during the next four years. While our lot was hard, we did consider ourselves fortunate in being able to keep our farm while so many people in other areas of the country lost theirs. We often compared our good fortune to the people called "Okies," displaced farmers living a nomadic existence.

With my new role as breadwinner, the neighboring farmers with whom we shared work began treating me as a man rather than a boy. That summer after my father's accident, at the completion of a job, I learned to smoke a pipe as well as roll Bull Durham cigarettes.

Things I learned in high school agricultural classes came in handy. Mending harnesses and fly nets, cleaning seed grain to get rid of the weed seed, and repairing worn-out and broken pieces of farm equipment, added to the twice-a-day chores and the in-season farm work, kept us very busy.

Our family's economic instability paled in comparison to that of many less fortunate throughout the country. We read in the papers about bank failures elsewhere, as well as many farmers and homeowners losing their homes. Even though we had lost the western twenty acres of our farm and the three cows, we were glad for our relative security. We were as apprehensive as everyone else at the time of President Roosevelt's inauguration in March 1933. We were electrified with the first radio broadcast of an inaugural speech, hearing the president outline some of the proposals that he would bring to Congress in the next several months.

Lest my readers think I have an impossible memory, I must now confess vague recollections in this area have been reinforced by referring to an old *World Book Encyclopedia* left on our den shelves when our son, Charles, now a therapeutic radiologist, left for college.

While I recalled the essence of the panic, I did not remember the particulars of the banking panic starting about three weeks before Roosevelt's inauguration. The ensuing run on the banks by depositors ruined many banks. Certainly, I did not recall that the day before Roosevelt's inauguration more than five thousand banks went out of business. I knew he had declared a bank holiday but didn't know it was March 6, 1933, just two days after the inauguration. Our banks in

Beaver Dam remained solid, but they were closed as were all banks in the United States until Treasury Department officials could examine every bank's books.

Banks in good financial condition were to be supplied with money by the Treasury and allowed to reopen. Those found in doubtful condition were kept closed until they could be put on a sound basis. Many banks that had been badly operated never opened again. The president's declaration of a bank holiday restored the confidence of the people and ended the bank crisis. The country knew that if a bank reopened its doors, it was financially sound.

The fact that Roosevelt had four hundred and seventy-two electoral votes to fifty-nine for Hoover may have had something to do with the lack of political gridlock at the time. Even his worst detractors could never accuse Roosevelt of being indecisive.

Inaugurated on March 4, 1933, he declared the bank holiday March 6, and on March 9, Congress began a special session called "The Hundred Days." This session actually lasted ninety-nine days, March 9 to June 16, in which Congress passed such important laws as the Agriculture Adjustment Act (AAA), the Tennessee Valley Authority (TVA), and the National Industrial Recovery Act (NIRA).

On March 12, Roosevelt gave the first of his famous fireside chats, speaking to the nation by radio, explaining what action had been taken and what he planned for the immediate future.

I think Dale Carnegie must have had FDR in mind when he had students in one of his sessions emphatically say, as they pound a folded newspaper on the podium, "Give me a man who gets things done!"

Our family profited from one of the first federal relief programs, the Civil Works Administration (CWA) in the winter of 1933-34. This program lasted only a few months and was subject to a great deal of criticism because it seemed to be "made work." However, it did give people a feeling that they were not getting handouts but were earning what they were given.

I can't remember exactly how much I got through the program for my own labor and that of our two horses and wagon. After getting up at four in the morning to do the milking, I drove the horses and wagon about five miles to the Shaw Hill Road outside Beaver Dam. There for eight hours I helped chip away at both sides of a hill to widen the road. The frozen dirt and stones would be loaded in my wagon by other equally needy people without teams. I think between the team and me, I earned four and a half dollars for a day's work during that winter.

Some of my friends participated in the Civilian Conservation Corps (CCC), which operated from 1933 until 1942 doing flood control, forestry and soil conservation projects. Some of the contour farming mentioned earlier was actually started then. The forests being logged now in northern Wisconsin were cultivated and planted by the CCC "boys."

The Works Progress Administration (WPA) was active between 1935 and 1941, when it employed an average of two million workers annually.

Present day concerns regarding the Social Security System and its stability would not be necessary had the Social Security Act of 1935 not passed.

Some of today's problems relating to the flight of jobs could well have been avoided had the National Labor Relation Act of 1935, giving workers the right to bargain collectively, not passed. While the aim was to give workers a fair shake, excesses going beyond the intent to have "a chicken in every pot" led to reactive changes that were not good for either labor or management.

It is unfortunate that we, as individuals or corporations can't simply live according to the precepts of the Golden Rule. We certainly don't "do unto others as we would be done by."

A personal experience in the spring of 1943, as well as later observations, convinced me that unions were not all good. In 1943, while awaiting transfer to the Great Lakes Naval Station, I had taken a job as an inspector at a company making braces for airplane wings being produced for the war effort. Union representatives called to my attention that my pile of scrap exceeded that of anyone else in the department. When I pointed out obvious flaws which might lead to the death of people using the airplane, I was told it was none of my business. Beside that, I was told I was turning out too many pieces, making the rest of the employees look bad. If I didn't mend my ways, there would be consequences!

Fifteen to twenty years later, when American Motors was going through a series of strikes, patients told me that the same attitude prevailed in the unions representing the workers in those plants.

I am convinced that the excesses of both unions and businesses have contributed almost as much as professional politicians to the sorry state at which our nation has now arrived. We have forgotten that the cost of things go up whenever the cost of production, with the add-on costs of Social Security, taxes, and interest on investment, exceed the value of the goods produced.

7

"Peas, Corn and Harebrained Schemes"

I am not certain why my social security number was not issued until June 26, 1937, since the Social Security Act was passed in 1935 to provide unemployment relief and old age assistance. The back of the card indicates I was then employed by Central Wisconsin Canneries so it may be that, under a certain age, one was not required to have a card.

After the spring's work had been completed in 1933, Uncle Marvin Keil who was comptroller for Central Wisconsin Canneries, arranged for me to get a job at thirty-two and a half cents an hour working in the pea packing plant. I could leave the farm because a seventeen-year-old cousin of the family who hauled our milk, came up to Beaver Dam from Grant County looking for work. He was very happy to work at our farm for $17.50 per month, plus room and board.

Child labor laws were not then in effect. In one twenty-seven day period I averaged seventeen and three-quarter hours a day at the canning factory. This created a positive balance in the family finances, if not in my constitution. One morning as the sun was coming up, I fell asleep on my bicycle and rolled in the ditch.

The following year, after the pea-canning season was finished, Uncle Marvin arranged for me to get a job in the canning factory at Fox Lake. That cannery plant was also a part of Central Wisconsin Canning Company, soon to become a part of Green Giant. The Fox Lake plant, which canned corn then, was eight or nine miles from the home farm.

At that point, I bought an old coupe for fifteen dollars. The rumble seat was taken out and modified to accommodate two fifty-five gallon drums. Arrangements were made with Uncle Art Butterbrodt to pay for my gas and oil in return for bringing to his farm two drums of waste corn from the plant to feed his pigs. When my work day was completed, the drums were partially loaded with corn and then lifted onto my make-shift truck where the filling was completed with a shovel. I then drove the ten miles to Uncle Art's farm along Dodge County Highway A, backed up to the loading dock, rolled the barrels off and loaded the two clean barrels he had left there from the day before. I then drove home and went to bed for a few hours.

Even in those days one couldn't expect much of a car for fifteen dollars. Great care was necessary in driving because it had virtually no brakes. Fortunately, I had no serious accidents, although a few chickens didn't know I couldn't stop and met untimely ends.

The friends I made in the canning factory were mostly older men, with children, who had been laid off from jobs either at the local Weyenberg Shoe or Malleable Iron Range companies. When our potato crop was ready for harvest, a few of the men were happy to work for a dollar a day and two meals. We did

70

throw in a few extra potatoes for them to take home.

In 1933 we sold our bull and made arrangements with our next door neighbor to have his bull service our cows when they were in heat. Harry and I would lead a cow next door and, after she was bred, take her back home.

At that time, Central Wisconsin Canneries had a huge silo that, when opened, enabled two or three teams of horses hitched to wagons to enter through corridors separating stacks of silage. The silage, which smelled awful, was the dietary mainstay of the local farms' cattle for the few months it lasted. It was an added bonus to the farmers, who were paid for the vegetables they grew. All growers were entitled to a fair portion of silage, in proportion to the number of acres they had in peas.

A few years later, about the time that Green Giant took over Central Wisconsin Canneries, the silo was demolished and pea viner stations closer to the farms were established. At that time, trucks would convey boxes of peas to the canning factory for processing. The vines were left at the viner in silage stacks.

One of my first jobs in the canning factory was emptying the sixty-five pound wooden boxes, with screen bottoms, into hoppers. The vegetables were then conveyed to the washer and then through various processes, finally coming out on conveyors in the cans, which were stored until a less busy season permitted labeling.

At that time, executives of the factory would taste each day's production to test its quality. I am not sure that the taste method is still used, but I do know that in the 1950s and '60s, it was the way peas and corn were graded by officials at our local Jackson and Rockfield canning plants. I vividly recall treating the president of our Jackson canning factory many times for diverticulitis, an inflammation of a chronic intestinal condition, when he would swallow rather than spit out the corn he was grading. His wife, still active at the age of ninety, remains my patient, as does their younger son.

I recall that during my internship, the head of the Radiology Department at Milwaukee Hospital impressed on his students the necessity for people with diverticulosis (out-pouching of the bowel) to avoid nuts, seeds, popcorn, and mayonnaise! While not all people with diverticulosis have flare-ups of inflammation if they eat these things, most of the cases of diverticulitis I have seen can be traced to dietary indiscretions. Having recently learned that I have diverticulosis, thus far I have not had a problem with the prohibited foods.

It seems surprising that it has taken almost sixty years for sexual harassment in the workplace to be a matter of concern. As an innocent youth I observed, when fellow employees called it to my attention, one of the officials of the plant making amorous, suggestive approaches to one or another of the women working on the night shift. A short time later, we would watch them "disappear" for a half hour or so. Rumor had it that those cooperative women would have a few hours overtime added to their paychecks! The company was actually paying for the extra favor as well as condoning it!

My later concern about habituating drugs may have had its origin in observing the effects of the over-use of a nasal inhaler containing Benzadrine on the life of one of my foremen at the canning plant. He initially used it for sinus problems, then found it helped him stay awake.

Before I leave the canning factory narrative, I don't want to forget to mention the snow storm of 1936. State Highway 151 between Beaver Dam and Waupun was closed for several weeks. The only access to Beaver Dam was by a team and bobsled. Trips were made to town for either groceries for ourselves or silage for our cattle. The passing sleds packed layers of snow so high on the roads that if one stood on the floor of the sled box, one could look over the telephone wires along the road. When State Highway 151 was closed because of the snowstorm, my Uncle Art and Aunt Florence had several snowbound guests for a few days.

Among the guests was a Dr. Twohig of Fond du Lac, a surgeon who made periodic trips to Beaver Dam. He was stuck on his way home. For many years after I started practice in 1948, both Hartford and West Bend were served by surgeons from Milwaukee or Fond du Lac, both thirty miles away.

8

"Back to School"

A telephone call yesterday from Mrs. Elaine Riopelle Paul, who had been a classmate of my sister Marge, set off another string of warm memories of my school days. While we were boy and girl, ours was not the usual boyfriend-girlfriend relationship. Her father was a successful physician who died young, leaving a lot of uncollectible bills and a family of teenagers for his wife to raise. I was welcome in their home almost as one of the family. We shared philosophical discussions and dreams. Her two older brothers were around the same age as my brother Harry. They were members of the class of 1937 and graduated with me from high school.

At our fifty-fifth class reunion in June 1992, I had a nice visit with one of her brothers and learned that Elaine was still alive and reasonably well, living in Tomahawk, Wis.

Elaine's youngest brother lives in Menomonee Falls. He had sent her a copy of a local publication called *50 Plus*, containing an article describing my enjoyment of the practice of medicine since 1948. It would appear that both of us realized that our adolescent dreams came true, even though the odds seemed so great back in the mid-1930s.

Similar feelings had been shared weeks earlier with Marcella Dinkel Feutz, another close friend of my sister Marge. She came to a chili supper at our church with a cousin who had read the same article. Over the years I had been richly blessed with friends of both sexes, as well as caring family, both of the present and past generations.

Resumption of school in the fall of 1936 was not as traumatic as I had anticipated. Whether or not the teachers were influenced by my added maturity or whether I actually achieved the grades I was given, I graduated with good enough grades to be accepted into the University of Wisconsin for the fall of 1937. During both my fourth year of high school and the first semester of my freshman year at the university, I continued to help my father and Harry on the farm in my spare time.

As mentioned earlier, Mrs. Barton provided me with a small bedroom on the third floor of her rooming house, which was located on the corner of Johnson and Mills Streets, very close to the university campus. (All the houses on that block have long since been demolished.)

That first semester of college, I would hitchhike the forty-two miles home early Friday afternoon, work on the farm Saturday and Sunday, and hitchhike back early Monday morning. Instead of the laundry box, which so many students of that era mailed home, I carried my soiled clothes in an old suitcase. Mother and Grandma washed them and had them packed, ready for me to carry back to school. We saved quite a bit of postage.

We also saved a considerable amount of expenditure for

groceries since Mother and Grandma Albrecht would always send me back with a couple loaves of bread and some jam, as well as an occasional sausage and cheese. Mrs. Barton and I shared meals, which she prepared.

I still have my little red booklet in which I detailed the expenditures of my first three years at the university. This record included numerous ten and fifteen cent Coke and malted milk expenditures, as well as books, tuition and incidental expenditures — even dates. It also included clothing expenses.

As I recorded, my expense for the first year, 1937-38, was $336.85. For the second year, it was $446.26, and for the third year $608.95, excluding room and board, which I earned as a houseboy for Mrs. Barton and, later, Mrs. Howard.

When it became apparent that Harry and Dad no longer needed my weekend help for the farm work, I found various part-time jobs through the university's Student Employment Agency. These jobs included changing screen and storm windows, washing windows and sometimes helping homeowners with garden work.

One of the most strenuous jobs I had was digging a hole under an existing frame house so that the owner could put in a basement. I don't think building permits were thought of in those days. I worried about the possibility of the supporting posts, set under the beams across various portions of the flooring, giving way while I was on my hands and knees working the soil from beneath the house to the outside.

Washing dishes in a restaurant was a way of filling vacation time. I remember working one New Year's morning until four o'clock, then going home to my room to change into my new suit, coat, hat, overshoes and gloves, procured with overtime pay at my various jobs over the previous months. Proudly, I took a ten-cent cab ride to the outskirts of Madison instead of a my usual five-cent bus ride, and hitchhiked home to my assembled relatives for the New Year's Day get-together.

I wonder how many of my readers remember what gift they gave their mother the Christmas of 1937. Each time I go to the garage, I admire the still functional, but almost worn out, round card table, covered in brown leather, with its folding legs and five folding chairs. I procured the card table and chairs from the Jenks furniture Store on Monroe Street in Madison. The set was delivered to my mother a few weeks before Christmas by the Jenks truck at no extra charge. Bob and Sally Jenks were quality people for whom I enjoyed working, both in the store and delivering that year.

One of the most traumatic events of my life occurred on March 28, 1938. I had been home the Sunday before and, as usual, helped Dad and Harry with the evening chores. I thought nothing of it when Dad asked if I recalled some author having written something like "Green grows the grass above me."

My father had attended Wayland Academy, a private school in Beaver Dam, and had wide-ranging interests in literature, so I didn't recognize his question as the danger signal it turned out to be. I helped with the morning milking and hitchhiked back to Madison for my late Monday morning class.

Two days later, as I was taking a written exam in Bascom Hall, a secretary came to my class and had the instructor ask me to come to the office. There I was told to pick up the telephone. The voice on the other end was that of Uncle Marvin Keil who said my father was ill and that I should get home as soon as possible.

Needless to say, my instructor excused me. I went back to my room and made arrangements with a friend to take care of my jobs. I then hitchhiked home.

The family was gathered in the kitchen along with Uncle Jack, Aunt Dorothy and Uncle Walde, as well as Uncle Marvin Keil. Apparently, Uncle Jack had been elected to break the news to me because he had "a way with words."

He gave me more than the usual vigorous hugs and by the

tear-stained faces of Mother, Marge, Harry and Carol, I sensed the news was not good. It wasn't until we got out to the barn that Uncle Jack told me Dad was dead.

There apparently had been an increase in Dad's depression which had been much more apparent a few years earlier. Dad had been complaining to members of the family about the rabbits that were chewing bark off the orchard trees and had actually shot some in the preceding few days.

On my last visit home, I noticed the shotgun leaning against the base on which the milking machine was placed in the barn. Dad had made arrangements with the milk hauler to bring something back from town when he delivered the empty cans. This was to spare my mother the shock of finding him. The milk hauler found him lying on the floor, between the milking machine and the cooling tank in the milk room.

At the time, we preferred to think of it as an accident and postulated how logical it was that he would be careless in picking up the gun to shoot some rabbits he probably saw through the open barn door. The coroner, however, indicated it was a suicide rather than an accident, and church officials felt constrained to request that he have a home funeral rather than one in church. The double indemnity on his life insurance, of course, was refused by the insurance company.

The open coffin was placed in the bay window of the living room by the undertaker who had served the family for years. Family, neighbors and friends were very supportive. The night before the funeral, after everyone had left, we had a private prayer session with Mother, Marge, Harry and Carol. We pledged to each other continued family support, come what may.

Harry became the head of the family at the age of eighteen. Marge returned to Milwaukee Hospital to complete her third year of nursing school, and Carol returned to grade school. The Monday following the funeral, I returned to my life in Madison and picked up the pieces.

It was about this time that my good friend Bob Gollhardt, who shared one of the three small rooms on the third floor of the Barton House, convinced me to go to Bethel Lutheran Church, where I developed a closer relationship with Jesus Christ.

The next two years were relatively uneventful. Summer vacations were spent at home helping Harry and working in the canning factory. The following winter and spring were filled with school and odd jobs, some of which were less frequent than in the first year. I continued associating with osteopaths from the time I met Dr. Keller. He introduced me to the Harned Brothers who had an osteopathic clinic next to the Quisling Clinic on Gorham Street in Madison, across from Bethel Lutheran Church. Drs. Jack and Lewis Harned taught me a good deal during those premedical school days.

At that time, the University of Wisconsin Medical School had a quota of qualified students who were given four-year appointments, and another quota of somewhat less qualified students who received two-year appointments to the medical school. Many of the more qualified students from the select group of four-year appointments couldn't cut the mustard. Some of the more qualified in the two-year appointment group replaced those who dropped out. Whether the interruption in my medical school days because of the war was a blessing in disguise, or whether I might have earned a coveted four-year appointment is a moot question.

The school year of 1940–41 was actually the last year for my Bachelor of Science degree and the first year of medical school. Studies were increasingly difficult and the ongoing battle with draft officials drastically curtailed my ability to make my own way. So I borrowed about one thousand-five hundred dollars from my mother to finish the year.

I don't think I will ever understand how my professors of

anatomy, Dr. Sullivan, Dr. Mortonson and Dr. Mossman, could possibly have put up with my differing from their teaching, based on my experience with the various osteopaths I had learned from over the preceding years. Once, during a hands-on demonstration with cadavers, it was asserted that the strong ligaments on either side of the sacrum made the sacroiliac joint immovable.

I at least had the grace to ask for a private audience with my professors.

They were surprised when I told them that based on my personal experience, having had an unstable left sacroiliac since the fall in the barn in 1929, that at least in my case, my sacroiliac was a movable joint. From the informal teaching I had received from osteopaths, many other people had movable sacroiliac joints which I had personally manipulated. They allowed me to demonstrate the instability of my own joint.

I am not sure that I ever convinced them that it should be taught that the sacroiliac joint could be moved if sufficient stress tore the ligaments, but at least they didn't kick me out of medical school for raising the question.

Osteopaths were not then highly regarded by medical doctors. It wasn't until the 1960s that some physicians felt that manipulative therapy had a place in medicine. The current acceptance of osteopathic physicians into the mainstream of medicine was probably accelerated by the shortage of MD physicians in the '60s and '70s. Prior to that, it was considered unethical to associate or learn from osteopaths, or even practice manipulative therapy. In that sense, I was unethical since I continued to manipulate those patients who would benefit from it, and even referred some of the more difficult cases to osteopathic physicians, including my old mentor, Dr. Keller.
Times change!

Hopelessness and frustration affect people in different ways. For a time, Harry left home to live and work for Uncle Walde.

My sister Marjorie felt inferior as she went to school, having to wear hand-me-down clothes and dresses made by Grandma Albrecht or our mother. Carol remembers being proud that I, her big brother, had brought her a snowsuit from Sears Roebuck with my hard-earned money. I don't think I felt inferior, although I was one of the only two boys wearing a sweater instead of a suit coat for the 1929 Future Farmers high school yearbook picture.

Two or three nights a week were spent with Dr. Keller and his family as I was learning osteopathic techniques. From him, I also learned philosophy and religion with a different perspective than my Lutheran tradition.

My father's condition after his fall from the silo had gradually improved so that by the fall of 1936 it was possible for me to return to high school to complete my senior year. Many of the teachers who had helped me when I left school four years earlier were still around. Classmates were, of course, all new; but they made me feel welcome, even though I was more driven to achieve. Extracurricular activities were limited because of my need to help with the farm work after school.

A few years earlier, one of my harebrained ideas for making money almost ended in disaster. I had fancied myself being able to make my way through the University of Wisconsin, if I ever got there, by being a boxer. At the time, the university was nationally known for its boxing teams.

I scraped together enough money for a set of boxing gloves and a weight bag. Together with a heavy grain bag filled with straw and barley, I had these set up on the barn floor. A professional boxer, who once had been a contender for the national middleweight title, had a gym in Milwaukee and offered lessons. Rich's Grocery in Beaver Dam made a weekly trip to Milwaukee to get provisions, so I hitched a ride on the truck every week to take boxing lessons. I fancied myself a real contender.

During the winter of my senior year in high school, I thought I was ready for my first venture as a fighter. I drove the twelve miles to Waupun after chores. My opponent for the first fight, I later learned, had already fought in five or six bouts. He was a much better boxer than the "local yokel" he faced.

I have no recollection of exactly what happened, but was later told that after I landed a few insignificant blows, my opponent hit me on the point of my chin. My body described an arc and my feet actually rose to the level of the top rope of the ring.

The back of my head made a resounding thud as it hit the floor of the ring.

I was carried to the locker room where I recovered a measure of competence. I have no recollection of driving home. The next morning, I had bilateral black eyes as a result of the concussion. The black eyes as well as a severe headache lasted a few weeks and I decided there must be a better way of making a living while making my way through school.

An earlier attempt to get rich quick fared no better. My grandmother Albrecht had a favorite recipe for a lotion which kept chapped hands soft. With the help of a friendly pharmacist, Ray Langmack, we had some labels made, he sold me some bottles and we went into production. A few relatives bought some, and the pharmacist possibly sold as many as six or eight of the twelve bottles he took as a courtesy. The remaining bottles soured and "Dew Drop Lotion" was allowed to expire.

One of the good experiences that has been beneficial to my patients over the years was getting acquainted, during my milking days, with Bag Balm. While this had been developed for farmers to use on the chapped teats and sore udders of cows, my family found that it was equally effective in keeping farmers' hands from chapping and cracking. During the years of my practice, while I haven't been able to prescribe Bag Balm, I have been able to suggest to pharmacists they carry some. I suggested to my farming patients, as well as some industrial patients, that if they asked the pharmacist for a little green square box of Bag Balm, which they could get for under five dollars, they just might save themselves the cost of a prescription drug, and would be able to use it for a year or two without consulting me again for a similar problem.

9

"Back to the Farm"

My experiences at Great Lakes Naval Station — my tour of duty, so to speak — and the war manpower pool as decreed by the local board, gave me an opportunity to observe the changes in farming between 1937 and 1943. More revolutionary changes in farming practices in Wisconsin and the nation have occurred in the last fifty years than in all the history of agriculture up to the days of the Great Depression. In many areas of Wisconsin, the chicken coops have long been unoccupied. Pig pens as we knew them in the '30s and '40s no longer exist, and in some areas, most barns are boarded up as one-family farms have yielded to corporate farming. The one-family farm is now the exception rather than the rule.

In 1943, farm workers were in short supply. I elected to work for a neighboring farmer, Willis Wendt, for thirty-five dollars a month and room and board, rather than for one of my well-to-do relatives.

Willis was a bachelor, and his father Ben was badly crippled with rheumatoid arthritis. Ben could no longer do any of the farm work, but could do the cooking.

During the next few months, I became involved in working with the youth and the Luther League at my old home church and, strange as it may seem, joined the choir which was badly in need of male bodies. Aunt Era Keil was the director. I think she questioned the wisdom of her appeal for choir members after I responded. For the rest of his life, my brother Harry laughingly referred to me as "Frankie" (as in Frank Sinatra). In later years, when my wife Marian was director of our choir at Christ Lutheran Church, she was happy that my professional obligations kept me from responding to her appeal for members!

Willis was still farming with horses, so my experiences of a few years earlier were pretty much duplicated while working for him. Despite rationing of gas and tires, Harry had converted pretty much to mechanized farming, although I believe he still had one team of horses.

The Ford truck we had mothballed in 1932 had been replaced by a more modern pickup and a heavy duty truck. Farmall tractors were then state-of-the-art and had replaced the horse-drawn equipment with which I was familiar.

Never again, except in memory, was I to enjoy husking corn with either a hook or a peg attached to my right hand: Grabbing the ear with my left hand, I would shuck off the covering with one swoop of the peg or hook; grabbing the ear of corn with my right hand, I would break it across the web between the thumb and index finger of my left hand; and with the same motion, throw it against the bang-board on the opposite side of the wagon box.

A well-trained team pulling the wagon responded to verbal commands to proceed forward after four or five rows of corn had been husked. Sometimes two or three corn huskers, each with his own row, almost made music with the rhythmic sound of the ears hitting the bang-board. At each end of the field, the horses had to be led or driven to the opposite side of the field, or turned around and the bang-board placed on the opposite side of the wagon box.

The corn had been planted in the spring with a two-row corn planter: Three or four kernels of seed corn in each "hill" about the same distance apart as the rows. This was accomplished by the tripping of a mechanism on the planter by the lumps on a tightly stretched wire running the length of the field. This wire had been unrolled from a reel on the planter prior to planting the field, and was rewound after the field was planted. Metal pegs at each end of the field held the wire taut. Each time the end of the field was reached, the operator got off the planter, moved the pegs and wire the appropriate distance to accommodate the next two rows. Corn to be used for silage was usually drilled rather than checked. The husking of corn became a bygone art as corn shredders were developed. At the time we are now recounting, corn pickers were becoming popular.

Marian recalls, two and one-half months after our marriage, riding in the wagon box and dodging corn cobs coming at her at a great rate of speed from the one-row corn picker pulled by the Farmall tractor driven by Bob Butterbrodt. Instead of sharing a ride with her on that beautiful, full-moon night, I was busy shoveling corn into the corn crib from a previously filled wagon.

I worked for Willis only a few months. Brother Harry's first marriage had gone sour and he joined the Navy. I returned home to help Bob Butterbrodt and Vilas King carry on with the work of the four farms.

Beside the farming, I felt the need to supplement our income by raising and butchering broilers. We still had the old hen house, but the major portion of the broiler operation was separate. Day-old chicks were bought at hatcheries and were raised on tiers of screen floors and fed with broiler food pellets procured from Hartzhein Seed and Feed, who in my prior role as a farmer had supplied us with feed for our livestock and sometimes with coal.

Neighboring farmers were happy to sell me very young roosters, and some of them were glad that I would come out in the evening and help catch the chickens while they were roosting in the trees after dark.

One night a week, three or four friends from town would come out after supper and we would spend several hours butchering, sometimes as many as two hundred broilers. As I recall, we cut them in half and delivered them to the refrigerators of our customers, which included The American Legion Hall, Rogers Hotel and local taverns. Chicken fries on Friday night have now been largely replaced with fish fries.

I shudder to think how brash I was; as I recruited customers, I told them, "If we ever deliver a defective bird, let me know, and I will eat it myself!"

A few months prior to our marriage on August 18, 1944, disaster struck when a fire of undetermined origin destroyed the building in which the broilers were being raised. Those not killed by the heat had to be destroyed by wringing their necks to put them out of their misery from chronic cough. That experience was probably responsible for my lack of enthusiasm about eating chicken, even to this day.

Our customers were notified that because of this disaster and the need to help Bob Butterbrodt and Vilas King operate Harry's farms during the time he was in the Navy, we would no longer be able to supply them with chickens.

10

"For Better
or for Worse"

D ecember 19, 1943, was one of the happiest days
of my life. My sister Carol was a freshman at
the University of Wisconsin during the World War II shortage
of housing in Madison. She had one of the five beds in a third-
floor dorm in the same Howard Lodge where six years earlier I had the basement room next to the furnace. One of her
roommates was Marian Peters from Bay View, a suburb of
Milwaukee.

For some reason, perhaps divine providence, I was elected
to pick Carol up for Christmas vacation. Somewhat later, I
learned that my little sister had confided in Marian and her
other three roommates, that she hoped her brother Harry
rather than Jim would pick her up. The idea behind that wish
was that Harry was much more responsible, and that Jim was

a maverick and an embarrassment. He didn't know what he wanted, and had had too many short-term girlfriends!

Some years later, that judgement was echoed by my cousin Edward Kellom when he and his wife visited us at our home in Jackson. I agreed with him wholeheartedly when he told Marian, in my presence, "Jim is lucky he got you. He never amounted to a hill of beans until he met you."

When I arrived in Madison, Marian and Carol took me to their meal co-op for supper. I remember driving back to Howard Lodge to drop Marian off before Carol and I took off for Beaver Dam. I told her how pleased I was to meet her and that I hoped to see her again.

A few days later Carol indicated she had been asked to accompany a soldier stationed at Truax Field in Madison to a New Year's Eve party. She wasn't too enthusiastic when I suggested that I would call Marian (whose Milwaukee telephone number I had had the foresight to procure), and see if she would care to make it a foursome. It was a delightful evening. I was thrilled when I took the girls back to Howard Lodge and Marian responded favorably to my suggestion that I hoped to see her again soon.

Marian took quite a bit of ribbing from her roommates when the long distance phone calls from Beaver Dam became more frequent.

After several dates, I learned that Marian was taking part in a project through the university's Home Economics House to host parties for lonely servicemen stationed in the area. One night in April I had a dinner date with Marian, knowing that at nine o'clock she would have to go back to the Home Economics House for a party. While in retrospect it seems presumptuous, I had taken the precaution of buying a diamond ring two days earlier, estimating what would be the right size.

After dinner, we drove out to a park on Lake Wingra, over which the sun was just setting. I told her that I loved her and would like to marry her. I said I didn't believe in long engagements and would she accept my ring (Carol had already told her about the red-haired nurse who had kept the ring I had exchanged for my typewriter a few years earlier.)

Marian had several reasons why she shouldn't accept my ring, the main one being a reluctance to saddle me with an unhealthy girl, who probably had a short life expectancy because of a chronic pulmonary problem. I convinced her that I would like it if she would share with me whatever time God would grant us, and I would like to have her "branded" as mine before I took her back to the Home Economics House party, to which I was not invited. She said, "Yes."

Because of the advent of penicillin and other antibiotics, the few years we had hoped for reached forty-eight. She put up with me through thick and thin and almost single-handedly raised our three children during the years when the practice of medicine was a demanding mistress.

Shortly after our engagement, Marian was to accompany Carol home from school to meet our family. (This time Carol's wish was granted, since Harry had gone to get them.)

Just before they were to arrive, I had gathered about thirteen dozen eggs from the hen house. In my haste to get everything in proper order, I stumbled going down the outside steps to the cellar. Although no bones were broken, my dignity was sorely stressed as I rolled on the basement floor at the foot of the stairs in the scrambled eggs, thus necessitating a bath before the arrival of my betrothed.

Needless to say, that first supper with my family was spent with Marian and me getting a good deal of kidding from the family and hired men about my having "fallen for her."

My visit to meet her family a few weeks later was even more tense. Her father and mother understandably were concerned, not only about her engagement to a farm boy hoping someday to be a doctor, but wanting to marry their daughter within a few months. Their Christian charity was sorely tried during that weekend visit. They tried to have us put off marriage for a year or two. I forcibly exploded and said that if they didn't give their permission for an early marriage, they would surely reconsider if I got Marian pregnant.

Her mother was almost as volatile as I, but her father characteristically kept his cool. Subsequently they became good friends and I had an endearing relationship with her family as long as they lived. They apparently had the philosophy, "If you can't beat him, join him."

Before our marriage, I had introduced Marian to the principal of Beaver Dam High School. The school was in need of another home economics teacher, so she was hired. We thought we were well set. Little did we know I would be a farmer for only three and a half months more!

After her graduation in June 1944, Marian got a summer job in Milwaukee sealing seams in B17 engine covers. Milprint was a factory which made packaging for food products, but like other industries, was converted to wartime production. Her co-workers were friendly, but street-wise, sharing their views in salty shoptalk, a shocking experience for a bride-to-be!

Paul, the job supervisor, was a singer at local events and offered to sing at our wedding. He sang "O Perfect Love" very well and later helped scoop ice cream at our reception!

We were married at Marian's church, Bay View Bethel Evangelical, at 7 p.m., August 18, 1944. It was a simple wedding; Marian's cousin Pearl and my brother Harry were the attendants. During our wedding ceremony, an unexpected phenomenon occurred. Bright rays of sunshine suddenly broke through a large stained glass window, shining directly down on us as the benediction was pronounced.

The reception was held at Marian's home where wedding cake and ice cream were served.

I took a week off for a honeymoon trip along the Mississippi River and western Wisconsin. We had frequent picnics, preparing meals on a little propane gas stove. This whetted our interest in camping trips quite a few years later.

Our wedding provides an interesting comparison to weddings of today. Marian's dress was a simple white formal with puffed sleeves; it cost eleven dollars. A headpiece with a short veil was four dollars! The comparison with today's wedding costs shows a real contrast in priorities, as well as the economy over forty-eight years.

We had arranged for Uncle Herb Butterbrodt to remodel the large bedroom Harry and I had shared to accommodate two wardrobes with a set of drawers between them. After returning from our honeymoon, we settled in our one room, sharing the rest of the house with the family. Marian started teaching home economics at Beaver Dam High School and I resumed my farming jobs.

In a previous chapter I described the circumstances leading up to my return to medical school at 7:30 a.m., January 1, 1945. At that point we felt Marian would work for a few years, supporting me through medical school. The best laid plans of mice and men....

We found a large light-housekeeping room on Dayton Street in Madison, only a few blocks from the university. Mrs. Van Able, our landlady, allowed us to use the kitchen and the laundry. Marian drove down weekends to visit me and, on one of these weekends while doing laundry, had a hemorrhage and passed what pathologists thought was an early pregnancy. However, her monthly periods did not resume, and she began to put on weight.

Two months later, after she had won a badminton contest among the teachers at Beaver Dam High School, Marian told me her ankles had been itching ever since she had helped stamp down clothing into barrels destined for Russian World Relief.

The following week my ankles started to itch.

We went to a dermatologist, who was one of my teachers. He diagnosed scabies and recommended a weekend of treatment with a foul-smelling sulfur compound, which we were to apply to every nook and cranny of our bodies and leave on for twenty-four hours. There had been an epidemic of scabies at a shoe factory in Beaver Dam. Evidently some of the discarded clothing which Marian stamped down, barelegged (nylons were unavailable), carried the "bug!"

The dermatologist also recommended we see a gynecologist, and arranged for us to see Dr. Thornton, a lady doctor (relatively rare for those days).

As it turned out, Marian was pregnant with our daughter Lynn, who arrived two months early on August 27, 1945, weighing only four pounds. She was a twin, remaining from what we had thought was a complete spontaneous abortion six months earlier!

By that time, we were living in a flat on Gorham Street, which we had procured for thirty-five dollars a month in return for taking care of the furnace, shoveling walks and cleaning the stairways. Lynn was in an incubator for twenty-seven days, at a cost of $7.50 a day!

We had a breast pump operated with water pressure to pump Marian's breasts a couple of times a day. With my bicycle, I took the milk to the hospital, a distance of about two miles. On a rainy day, going up a hill on Gorham Street, I dropped the bottle; Lynn had to receive milk that day from another donor.

I shudder to think what the cost would be for twenty-seven days in an incubator now. Needless to say, our thoughts of Marian supporting me through medical school did not materialize. Despite this, we managed until my graduation in June 1947.

CHAPTER

11

"Tuberculosis"

Within a few months of the birth of our daughter, emotional tensions once again ran high when a routine tuberculin test was not only positive, it was so positive it produced a large crater in my right arm.

This infection undoubtedly was incurred during my time at Cleveland State Hospital when I was doing gastric aspirations on many of the patients. But knowing the probable source of the infection didn't do any good in allaying my apprehensions.

How was I to go about getting through medical school and support a wife and daughter? While Marian could teach, it didn't seem right for her not to be a full-time mother.

As the tuberculous lesion in my right upper lung was being observed, there was really a great deal of emotional tension as we wondered when and if Dr. Helen Dickey, who probably knew more about tuberculosis than anyone else in Wisconsin, would tell me to quit medical school and go to a sanatorium. We were relieved when she elected to let me stay in medical school, but said I could do no outside work. Three series of daily gastric aspirations were all negative, so it was assumed I was no danger to others and that the lesion was already encapsulated.

The dramatic changes noted earlier in agriculture are paralleled or exceeded by the changes in medicine during my lifetime.

Prior to the mid-1930s when sulfonamide became available, death rates from infectious diseases were horrendous. Many people, including Marian, developed sensitivity to the early forms of sulfonamide. Newer forms of sulfonamide with less toxicity were available and instrumental in preserving the lives of our servicemen from both wounds and illness in World War II. There was a significant reduction in mortality as compared to servicemen of World War I. All age groups in the civilian population were similarly blessed.

While Alexander Fleming discovered penicillin in 1928, it wasn't until almost twenty years later that it became widely available for clinical use. An effective drug treatment for tuberculosis was still another fifteen or twenty years away. Even in the first few years after I started practicing medicine in 1948, I had numerous patients with pulmonary tuberculosis who were sent to sanatoriums for rest until they were no longer a hazard to others.

Dr. Dickey continued to observe me closely. When the lesion began to regress and I was able to continue in medical school, I began to feel more comfortable.

While I was at the medical school at Wisconsin, senior students were expected to spend some time in training outside of Madison, including two weeks at the sanatorium at Wales, Wis. I will never forget the look on Dr. Dickey's face when I asked whether I couldn't be excused from this portion of my education for fear I might get tuberculosis again. In her gruff voice, she looked at me with only a trace of a smile and said, "Albrecht, if you ever die of tuberculosis, it will be from what you already have and not from what you get as a new infection."

I still have a few patients who have scars from the last-ditch surgery for tuberculosis and empyema (pus in the lungs) resorted to when the generally prescribed rest and hygiene treatment of that era failed to let their bodies conquer those diseases.

It is almost impossible to understand how in such a relatively short time the therapeutic "ball game" has changed. For many years now, drug treatment has diminished the need for sanatorium care and most people can be treated at home. None of the sanatoriums of the past are currently in operation. The old Wales Sanatorium, where I spent two weeks for training after being persuaded to go by Dr. Dickey, is now a state juvenile prison. This may well change if current trends of resistant germ strains and people's resistance to the recommended regular use of proper medicine continues. Recently, the question has been posed as to whether the AIDS epidemic might cause such a reversal in the treatment of tuberculosis again.

I mentioned earlier Marian's reluctance to marry me because of a life-long battle with repeated sinus infections, pneumonia and chronic lung disease. She also had severe allergies which contributed to the promotion of infections. I suggested we put it in God's hands. He has richly blessed us, as well as all humanity, with the development not only of penicillin but with the newer more specific antibiotics and advances in the treatment of allergies.

The last six months of my senior year of medical school were to be spent outside Madison. Therefore, we moved our meager possessions to Milwaukee to live with Marian's parents while I was on clinical rotation. Marian and our daughter Lynn lived there and I visited between assignments. That spring

Marian developed pneumonia and spent two weeks at Milwaukee Hospital under the care of Dr. Einar Daniels, receiving what today would be considered infinitesimal doses of 25,000 units of penicillin intravenously every three or four hours, for nearly two weeks. At that time, hospital committees decided which patients received the limited amount of penicillin available.

As I look at the old picture of "The Doctor" on the wall above my desk, I am humbly grateful for Grandma Albrecht. So many years ago she taught me perseverance when she said, "Jimmy, not *if* you get to be a doctor, but *when* you get to be a doctor." She promised that when I became a doctor, the picture would be mine. I can still see her walking across Camp Randall Stadium with the picture in a brown paper bag that June day in 1947 when I received my medical degree.

I am also grateful for having lived through and, to some extent, participated in the thrilling advances of medicine during my lifetime. We have been deeply blessed!

12

"The Last Years of Medical School and Internship"

In the spring of 1946, coinciding with the apparent stabilization of my tuberculous lesion, I was giving chloroform anesthesia to a dog my classmates were to perform surgical procedures on, when the "patient" regurgitated and died of anoxia (oxygen deprivation) from the foreign material in his lungs.

Our instructor, Dr. Orth, took the opportunity to let me and the other students on my team know that many people were dying in the same way because inadequately trained people were giving them anesthesia.

While my patient that day was only a dog, a temporary depression led me to Dr. Ralph Waters at University Hospital, one of the first anesthesiologists in the United States and, earlier in life, a physician in Kansas. He had lectured to our junior medical class on one occasion and had appealed to me as the type of physician I would like to be.

Dr. Waters listened to me as I told him my dream of becoming a family physician. But being eight years older than my classmates, I told him, I wouldn't have time to get formal training in anesthesia before starting practice after my internship. I had to support my family.

After my experience with the dog, I wanted to be prepared to avoid the same thing happening to any of my patients. I asked Dr. Waters for help. From the smile on his face, I could tell the answer was going to be positive. He told me that he would have to talk to his residents and that I should come back in a few days to see if they could work something out.

That bad experience with the dog turned out to be a blessing in disguise, as have many experiences in my life. Dr. Waters and the anesthesia residents arranged a unique preceptor arrangement. In return for my maintaining the anesthesia machines at University Hospital, Dr. Waters and his residents would each teach me the area of his expertise. They all knew I didn't intend to become an anesthesiologist, but wanted the experience to make me a more competent family physician. Little did we know that from 1948 until 1975, I would be both.

I learned both oral and nasal intubation from Dr. Noel Gillispie, who had written a book on the subject; the techniques of spinal anesthesia from one of the residents; block anesthesia from another; and the dangers of local anesthesia improperly administered from a third. Dr. Waters himself taught me inhalation anesthesia with cyclopropane, and another resident taught me the techniques of good ether anesthesia. Pre- and post-operation rounds with one or more of my mentors were an added bonus, supplementing the advice of my professors on the necessity for adequately documenting both positive and negative observations. In those days, such documentation was considered necessary for the good of the patient. The documentation also furthered the understanding of the intern following up on the medical student who, in those days, was the first to evaluate patients entering University Hospital, referred there by an LMP (local medical physician). The record became substantial as the resident in that department of the hospital added his observations to that of the medical student and intern.

The attending physician or surgeon expected each medical student to accompany him on rounds to each of the patients we worked up. We were expected to be prepared to discuss reasons for our conclusions in establishing a diagnosis. It is unfortunate that in the last several years such adequate documentation is probably considered more important for the protection of the doctor from malpractice suits than it is for the good of the patient.

My extracurricular activity working with the anesthesiologists, in addition to full-time medical school, gave Marian a sample of what life would be like for the years ahead.

As a junior and senior medical student, for a few days between the departure of one intern and the arrival of another, I was permitted to act as an intern, making pre- and post-op rounds and ordering pre-anesthetic medication, with the senior resident giving final approval.

My experiences in my final years of medical school were important to my future out of all proportion to what I had anticipated when I enlisted Dr. Waters' help.

Anesthesiologists in 1947 and 1948 were in short supply. Dr. Bookhammer and Dr. Beffel were anesthesiologists at Milwaukee Hospital, where I served my internship. Dr. Wilson Phillips was at Mt. Sinai Hospital in Milwaukee. Nurse anesthetists did the bulk of anesthesia at both hospitals, with the MD anesthesiologist generally taking the more difficult cases, where complications could be expected.

While my internship did not include an official rotation

through anesthesiology, Dr. Bookhammer and Dr. Beffel took me under their wings in the same manner Dr. Waters and the residents at University Hospital had. Even while on other rotations during my internship, I learned something about anesthesia from them.

Toward the end of my internship, Dr. Bookhammer suggested that since I was going to be practicing in nearby Jackson, I might wish to work for him as well, giving anesthesia at Milwaukee Hospital until I got my practice established.

There were several reasons why I eventually agreed. First, there was a hiatus from June 1, when I completed my internship, to the middle of August, when I expected to hear whether I had passed the State Board exam. I also could assume that it would be several more months before my fledgling practice would earn enough to support Marian, Lynn and, by then, another baby on the way. It seems incredibly fortunate to me that Dr. Bookhammer was willing to pay me $800 a month out of his own pocket just to further my education.

At that time of change for hospitals, from a reliance on nurse anesthetists to a reliance on MD anesthesiologists, with the latter being in short supply, there were varying opinions as to the place for each.

Dr. Bookhammer wanted me to have the experience of working with Dr. Phillips at Mt. Sinai, and he arranged for me to be there for two weeks. Dr. Phillips had the conviction that an anesthesiologist had the obligation to use his expertise for the benefit of all patients in the hospital. As a consequence, he supervised five or six nurse anesthetists. At that time, nurse anesthetists had not yet acquired the skills to intubate patients. Therefore, he would be available while "putting the patient to sleep" and at the proper time, when anesthesia was sufficiently deep, do the intubation. When he saw that everything was going smoothly, he would go to the next room. If any problems arose, he was available to help solve them. It kept him busy.

Until my license arrived on August 6, 1948, I drove to Milwaukee Hospital or Mt. Sinai early every morning and worked until the day's schedule was completed. After the arrival of my license, until October of that year, I continued going to the Milwaukee hospitals each morning, and had office hours in Jackson from one until six o'clock daily. Saturday mornings my office hours were from eight in the morning until twelve. Every Monday, Wednesday and Friday evening, I had office hours from seven until we finished.

Both St. Joseph's Hospital in West Bend, eight miles north of Jackson, and Hartford Hospital, west of Jackson, had nurse anesthetists who were Catholic nuns. Initially I had acquired my knowledge of anesthesia only to help my own patients. But I suppose my few weeks with Dr. Phillips had something to do with my decision that God wanted me to spread myself even thinner for the good of a greater number (to the further detriment of my family obligations). I helped out at both hospitals.

Dr. Bookhammer proposed me as candidate for the Wisconsin and American Society of Anesthesiologists. Initially, I was a junior member, and then an active member until 1975. I am currently a retired member. Actually, I was a member of the Society of Anesthesiologists some months before I became a member of the Academy of Family Practice.

By October 1948, with the help of Dr. Bookhammer, I had a made-to-order anesthesia machine delivered to St. Joseph's Hospital in West Bend, while the Sisters at Hartford bought a machine to my specifications. The two nurse anesthetists at both hospitals wanted to retire, but they kept on doing the obstetric anesthesia and some of the simpler cases. For a number of years I spent three mornings a week giving anesthesia at Hartford and three mornings giving anesthesia at West Bend.

In the spring of 1953, by which time I was coroner of Washington County, I developed an orchitis, an infection of my testicles, after I was struck by a towing cable attached to a car demolished by a train, two miles south of Jackson. The car's driver required my services as a coroner rather than a doctor, and I ended up in the hospital as a patient for a week. Another several weeks of convalescence necessitated arranging for a locum tenens, a temporary substitute, to cover my practice while I recovered.

I owe Dr. William C.P. Hoffman of Hartford, another family doctor, a debt of gratitude for coming over to my office to keep my family practice intact during those weeks until Dr. Harry Evans arrived to fill in. I taught Dr. Evans enough of the principles of anesthesia that in 1955, he decided to become an anesthesiologist himself.

When I recovered, once again I spread myself too thin. Ultimately, Hartford Hospital arranged for its own anesthesia coverage, so I no longer had that obligation.

While I remained head of the department supervising nurse anesthetists at the West Bend hospital until 1975, I devoted much less time to anesthesia after about 1965.

13

"On to Graduation"

The Preceptorship Program at the University of Wisconsin required some time away from Madison during the senior year. My out-of-town experiences were planned for the last part of the year so that we could save money by having Marian and Lynn live with her parents in Milwaukee while I was on these assignments.

I think it was in early December 1947, when we moved from Madison to the Peters' home in Bay View, with my first assignment as an extern at St. Mary's Hospital in Wausau, Wis., nearly 200 miles to the north. There I made the acquaintance of the Sisters of the Divine Savior, the same order with whom I worked in later years at St. Joseph's Hospital in West Bend. They also had small hospitals in Columbus and Portage, Wis.

I no longer remember whether my externship at St. Mary's

Hospital was a two- or three-month assignment, but many things happened there that have stuck in my memory, over and above the loneliness of being away from my family.

Within a week or two of my arrival in Wausau, I incurred the displeasure of one of the medical staff. The doctor had admitted a patient with a sore throat to a ward in the hospital, just prior to the doctor's leaving for a football game in Madison, one hundred and forty miles away. Before he left, he wrote the appropriate orders for the treatment of a streptococcal sore throat.

As I examined the patient, I was impressed with a mouse-like odor which Dr. Middleton, one of my university professors, once had described as being characteristic of diphtheria, which was no longer common in Wisconsin. The appearance of the patient's pharynx coincided with the description of the diphtheritic membrane. The slide I made and stained with the help of the nun lab technician suggested to both of us that this indeed was diphtheria. (The patient had recently returned from duty in Europe where diphtheria was still a problem.)

On the basis of this, I spoke to the Sister Superior at the hospital and suggested the patient be moved to a private room and precautions taken to protect others until we had a definite diagnosis. In the meantime, we called a branch of the State Lab in Stevens Point and a courier took our slides there, together with a fresh specimen.

My diagnosis was confirmed, but the attending physician, when he returned from the football game, was less than appreciative of my being responsible for putting his patient in a private room!

The hospital's chief of staff appreciated my decisiveness, though, and wanted to teach me to be a surgeon. (It was still possible for people to get to be specialists by the preceptor method in those days.) His office staff nurse did not share his enthusiasm and discouraged the idea, so that a few months later he reneged on that invitation. I felt then, as I do now, that God was directing my path according to His wishes, if not mine at the moment.

Many of the nuns I met at St. Mary's Hospital later worked with me at St. Joseph's Hospital in West Bend. I still have the notebook in which I wrote down recipes for various ointments as prepared by the German nun, Sister Winnebalda, at St. Mary's. Gerald Baum, a classmate who shared the rotation at Wausau, eventually became, as I found out at the time of our thirty-fifth class reunion, a pulmonary specialist in Israel. While at Wausau, he taught me to tie a perfect knot in the tie all self-respecting physicians were expected to wear.

Two weeks with Dr. Max Fox at the Contagious Disease Hospital on Mitchell Street in Milwaukee allowed me to share some time with my family. The rotation in Chicago at the Chicago Lying In Hospital acquainted me with the big city side of life my farm background had not really prepared me for.

The experience of living in an old Chicago jail for our protection, making pre- and postpartum calls, and delivering babies in squalid tenement houses were unique experiences for me. This introduced me to a way of life I had not previously known. Predominantly, we worked with underprivileged Blacks, Mexicans and Gypsies.

Usually two of us went out on each assignment. When a woman was in labor, we would stay with her during the course of labor until the baby was delivered. If there were complications, we would call for help and she would be transferred to a hospital. On one occasion, as a man came up the stairs, I asked the lady who had just delivered whether I should show the baby to her husband. I couldn't believe it when she just smiled at me and said, "He ain't my husband. He's my boyfriend!"

Another, more tense, situation developed as we prepared to deliver a Gypsy lady. We had all of the boiled water ready, the instruments sterilized, and were waiting for the arrival of the baby in the presence of quite a large number of the tribe. We became apprehensive when we saw the husband stroking a knife, letting us know we had better not goof up. We didn't!

One of my fellow students from Madison, on his way home from a delivery just outside our jailhouse home, was accosted by two people who demanded his money. After he had given them his wallet, they slit the back of his pants and used his dropped pants to hobble him as they took off. I can truthfully say that none of my experiences in Jackson have been as exciting.

A rotation in Chicago's Cook County Hospital was another experience to prepare students for their future lives as doctors.

We all gathered in Madison for final exams and graduation, final good byes and well-wishes to classmates, many of whom we would never see again. Some did not return for any of our reunions.

One of the differences between then and now is the relatively small percentage of women doctors. I think our class had only three!

I find it hard to understand why it has taken society so long to accept women physicians, although I expect such sexual discrimination has not been limited to the medical profession. Certainly, the women physicians with whom I have been associated have been well-qualified, caring individuals, into whose hands I would entrust my loved ones or myself.

14

"Introduction to Jackson"

Early in my internship, in the fall of 1947, we realized I couldn't afford any more time in training. In those years many doctors started practice with only one year of internship for their postgraduate training.

Some of my family would have liked us to go back to Beaver Dam, or at least to nearby Fox Lake, which might have been a good opportunity for us. But Marian and I knew there was some truth in the statement Jesus had made some nineteen hundred years earlier, "A Prophet is not without honor, except in his own country." We realized that my past record as a farmer and conscientious objector might be a disadvantage in starting a practice in my old home town.

Marian's uncle, Elmer Kleffen, was a field man for Luick Dairy Company (now part of Sealtest). He was well acquainted with the farmers in the Jackson area. He was also acquainted with some of the businessmen of Jackson, which had lost its physician, Dr. Froede, to the war effort in 1943. Two of Uncle Elmer's Jackson area friends, Harold and Edna Hoefert, who were just getting established in farming, and the widowed Andy Loduha, had told him how Jackson had always had a doctor until 1943.

Two business people in Jackson, both now deceased, Melvin Gumm of Hoge & Gumm General Store, and Ort Butzke, who owned Butzke Electric and Implement, as well as a local Chevrolet dealership, impressed on Uncle Elmer how much they did need a doctor and how much a doctor would mean to the surrounding population of farmers who regarded Jackson as "the center of the universe — between Kirchayn and Katzabach!"

Marian's folks were delighted at the prospect of having their daughter and granddaughter — and I think, by that time, even their son-in-law — living within thirty miles of Milwaukee. My mother, stepfather and Harry's family lived in Beaver Dam, forty miles west of Jackson.

Arrangements were made for us to meet with the Jackson Village Board in the middle of the week between Christmas and New Year's Eve. While a Village Board meeting was not scheduled until seven in the evening, we drove out early enough to explore the village and surrounding area.

Years later, Marian remembered that the sign at the west entrance of the village listed a population of 361. We were greatly impressed with the civic pride evidenced by the beautiful Christmas decorations on the main street. We also were delighted with the warm reception we received from the local undertaker, H. B. Woldt, and his wife when we stopped at their home to ask permission for Lynn (and us) to use their bathroom before proceeding to the Village Hall, where we were to meet with the Village Board. It appeared that everyone in this small town was pulling for the Village Board "to make the sale" with the new doctor.

Recently, I had the pleasure of visiting with the only surviving member of that Village Board, John Indermuehle, and his wife at a local restaurant. We shared warm memories of that night of long ago. It seems impossible now, when one considers the current one hundred thousand dollar salary needed by a young doctor starting out, that as the five members of the board told me about the wonderful potential of Jackson, I asked with some trepidation whether they would be able to guarantee I would have a *gross* income of twenty-five hundred dollars my first year. If they would, I would agree to come for one year.

All five board members agreed, and we shook hands on the deal. They were to arrange for us to have an apartment, at a fair price, ready for us to move into by June 1. They were also to arrange for the tenants who had made an apartment out of Dr. Froede's old office to leave by June 1.

The old doctor's office was on the east side of a large house then owned and occupied by Lester Klumb and his wife Evelyn. Lester was manager of the Jackson Canning Factory, which was a subsidiary of the Rockfield Canning Company, owned by the Klumb family. Two years later Mr. Klumb would sell the house to us.

The week after meeting with the Village Board, an incident occurred that made me question the wisdom of our decision to move to Jackson.

One of my patients at Milwaukee Hospital, Mrs. Paulus of Cedarburg, asked me to stop at her room after my full day as an intern. It came as no surprise when she said, "Dr. Albrecht, I like you!"

I responded, "I like you too, Mrs. Paulus."

"That wasn't the reason I asked you to come to see me," she stated. "My father had been the doctor at Grafton. Grafton no longer has a doctor, and I would like to establish a memorial to him. I will set you up with a home and an office, rent free, as a memorial to my father."

Grafton was a larger village just ten miles east of Jackson, adjacent to Cedarburg in Ozaukee County.

I was almost speechless after hearing her offer. Finally, I said, "Mrs. Paulus, why didn't you talk to me last week?"

She asked why, and I stated, "Just a week ago last night, I told the people of Jackson that I would come out there."

"Do you have a contract?" she asked.

"No," I said. "But my word is my contract. We shook hands on the deal."

She said, "I can understand that. Why don't you just plan on staying the year you agreed and then come to Grafton?"

My reply was that in the event we didn't make the twenty-five hundred dollar guarantee, I would feel free to accept her offer. In reality, I expected that within a year Grafton would have a physician, and, indeed the community did.

As it turned out, the Jackson Village Board members were right. Not only did we exceed the gross income of twenty-five hundred dollars, but we exceeded that with net income as well.

Mrs. Paulus remained my friend until her death several years ago. There was always a February birthday card as well as a pleasant smile and a little discount when I stopped at her meat market in Cedarburg from time to time over the years.

When I finished my internship on June 1, we settled in the four-room lower flat the village had arranged for us to rent. It was located a block west of the railroad tracks that bisected the village, on the north side of Main Street. We became acquainted with our neighbors and the other town people. We joined Christ Lutheran Church, which was then situated between the two-room elementary school and the Woldt Funeral Home. (During the next year the church was moved to its present location on the east end of the village, where a basement had been dug to provide an added Sunday school room, Fellowship Hall and kitchen.)

While waiting for my medical license to arrive, my mornings were spent going to Milwaukee Hospital to give anesthesia under the direction of Dr. Bookhammer. My afternoons were spent getting equipment and furniture for my office. One narrow room, which had been a pantry, became my drug room and laboratory. What had been the bedroom for the previous tenants became my main treatment room. What had been a small living room was my waiting room. Between the waiting room and treatment room was an office in which I had a big desk and chair, as well as an old-fashioned, green plush couch against the wall opposite my desk. On that wall I had a large map of Washington County which would enable me to quickly find my way to the farm homes I soon would be called on to visit.

My practice, once composed of perhaps ninety percent farming people and ten percent village residents, changed by the mid-1970s to perhaps one percent farm people and ninety-nine percent people who made their living in urban business and industry. Currently, I doubt if as much as .005 percent of my practice is made up of actively farming people.

During June, July and early August, I spent my mornings at Milwaukee Hospital giving anesthesia, and my afternoons planning and arranging my little office. We had procured some supplies and equipment during my internship, based on what various doctors I met suggested I would need to be well equipped. Some of the family doctors told me what surgical instruments I would need to do tonsilectomies and adenoidectomies. Obstetricians gave me advice on what dilators and gynecological equipment, including speculum, ring forceps and head mirrors, I would need. Laryngoscopic equipment, both for direct and indirect laryngoscopy, were a must, not only for my anesthetic practice, which was to develop in October, but also for use on someone choking on a foreign object.

Right from the start, I carried blankets and oxygen in the trunk of my car. Fortunately, I didn't have to use them until after I got my license. I think if any event demanding the use of oxygen had come to my attention, I probably would have taken a chance on practicing medicine without a license, hoping that the Good Samaritan theory would save me. To my good fortune, I never had to test that theory.

I did take one boy with an obvious hip problem along with me to Milwaukee one day in June or July to see one of the orthopaedic men, who corrected a malrotation of the boy's hip. Subsequently, after I had been in practice for some years, the boy's other hip was operated on, as well.

15

"Start of Practice
— August 1948"

Many times, Marian and I wondered how we could have possibly had enough faith that I would pass my state board exam four weeks after we moved, and that we would be able to continue paying the thirty-five dollars a month rent on our flat and thirty-five dollars a month for my small office. Knowing we had the anesthesiology job to rely on until I passed the exam that would enable me to practice medicine may have played a part in our acting "as fools where angels fear to tread."

At any rate, I did pass the state boards. What an embarrassment it would have been had I failed!

August 6, 1948 was a red letter day. On my usual stop at the post office, there was a fellow named Harold sitting on the steps. "I am your first patient!" he announced.

Harold had broken his arm four hours earlier and had gone to the post office to ask the post master if Doc's license had arrived. When informed that an official looking letter from Madison was there for me, and on holding it to the light it appeared to have a certificate inside, Harold elected to wait until "Doc" got back from Milwaukee so he could be my first patient.

On opening the envelope in the presence of the post master and Harold, we were all elated to find I could officially take care of my first patient without fear that I'd be practicing medicine without a license.

I splinted his arm and took Harold to St. Joseph's Hospital in West Bend where I had already been granted staff privileges. We obtained an x-ray to confirm the obvious diagnosis and consulted with Dr. Raymond Frankow of West Bend. Dr. Frankow had honored me some months earlier when he came to Milwaukee Hospital one day, after learning that I was going to establish a practice in Jackson. He offered his support, friendship and help when I needed it. Dr. Frankow helped me with the cast that day and, with his partner, Dr. A. T. Grundahl, we had an agreeable association, mutually helping each other over many years until they both retired.

By the time I got back to Jackson and had lunch, several other people had learned by word of mouth that "Doc's" license had arrived. I saw them at the office and my practice was off to a flying start.

On the weekend before the arrival of my license, many relatives from Milwaukee and Beaver Dam gathered at my office to assist Marian and me in addressing envelopes and announcements to all the people listed in the telephone books of the Jackson, Slinger, West Bend and Cedarburg areas. These ready-to-go announcements were taken to the post office and mailed first class the same day my license arrived.

The announcements included our name and address, 118

Main Street, Jackson, Wisconsin (no Zip Code then), phone number and office hours. The office phone number was 85W and our home phone number was 85R. Many years later, even after our telephone numbers had long since changed, I would find these announcement cards posted on the telephone or the wall next to the telephone in many of the farm homes where I made home visits.

My active staff membership application for practicing medicine, surgery and anesthesiology had been prepared and submitted to the medical staff of both the West Bend and Hartford hospitals, with the request they be approved conditional on my receiving my license. The same day I received Wisconsin doctor's license number 10270, it was given to the Mother Superior at each hospital. Each Mother Superior then informed the chief of staff at each hospital and I was able to admit patients. Similar arrangements at Milwaukee Hospital enabled me to directly admit patients there.

As my workload in Jackson, West Bend and Hartford increased, my anesthesia work at Milwaukee Hospital decreased. Between the middle and the end of October I discontinued practicing anesthesiology in Milwaukee entirely, except for one brief period a few years later when St. Luke's Hospital was built at its current location on Oklahoma Avenue. One of the surgeons who came to Hartford, Dr. Adamkiewicz, invited me to come to the new, big city hospital and consider limiting my practice to anesthesiology. While things went well from the anesthetic standpoint, the close to an hour trip to and from St. Luke's made it obvious that should I accept the invitation, it would mean changing directions and becoming less than the family physician I had felt called to be. I declined the St. Luke's offer.

Nonetheless, I continued to spread myself too thin trying to be all things to all people, until I finally retired from anesthesiology. In 1975 I became a nondues-paying, retired member of the Wisconsin and American Society of Anesthesiologists.

Prior to moving to Jackson, part of my intern responsibilities had been serving the needs of patients at the Martha Washington Home for unwed mothers, some distance from Milwaukee Hospital. One of the girls in the home had not adjusted well to group living and was in need of some financial support. By that time, Marian was expecting our second child, Peter, due to arrive September 27, 1948. It seemed appropriate to offer this girl the opportunity of living in a private home in return for helping to get home and office ready. I can't remember if she received any stipend beyond room and board and spending money.

Between the time we moved to Jackson on June 1 and August 16, 1948, the day my license arrived, we had cleaned and equipped the office and examining room with furniture and instruments from medical supply houses in Milwaukee.

Shortly after starting practice, it became apparent that I would need help. I made arrangements to hire the first of many loyal assistants. Virginia Gilbert was working at Gumm's store. She had recently lost her husband, and seemed to be the type of person I needed to help me get acquainted with the community, as well as to run my office.

Mel Gumm hated to lose her, but felt obligated to help out the young doctor he had agreed to subsidize if things didn't go well.

Virginia Gilbert became my first office girl and medical assistant. She got me off to a good start and remains a good friend to this day. She left my employ in 1953 after she married Elroy Borchert and started raising their family. Virginia was the first of a long line of dedicated employees who were largely responsible for enabling me to serve the needs of the area's growing population in an era when doctors were in short supply.

With the office having gone through a total of nineteen major and minor alterations in the interval from 1948 to 1983, some of my aging recollections may not be quite accurate. In the days of my youth and middle age, any need that was apparent was addressed forthwith without the need for prolonged committee discussions.

Today, most young doctors starting in established clinics don't have to furnish and equip their offices and treatment rooms. Things were different then.

During my internship tour of duty in the Ear, Eye, Nose and Throat Department, I bought a special surgical lamp to provide light for the tonsillectomies I did as an intern, under the guidance of EENT specialists. Subsequently it served as a surgical light in my office for well over thirty years. Many used instruments were procured from some of the older family practice physicians who were winding down their practices and no longer doing deliveries or tonsillectomies. A water suction apparatus, as well as sinus irrigation equipment, were a must. A plain, four-legged table of the proper height for treating back patients fit in the narrow combination drug room and lab, which also accommodated an infrared lamp.

One night, about two in the morning, Dr. Keller, my old mentor, stopped on his way back to Beaver Dam from Milwaukee. While treating me on my new table, we decided the table was too high so we set out to lower it to the right height.

While we had a square and a saw, neither of us were accomplished carpenters. The legs were sawed off in increments before the table was level. Dull saw and hard wood, perhaps? It ended up being a little shorter than we had planned. The next morning, our neighbors in the house to the east inquired about the sawing heard during the night.

On the shelves above this auxiliary treatment table were stock bottles of various medications that didn't fit in the former kitchen's cupboards, located above the long sink and countertop. For the first four and one-half years of my practice, I dispensed medications, as did most of the doctors in those days.

We changed to prescribing medications for reasons I'll explain later.

Secondhand furniture was acquired for the small waiting room. The corridor leading from the waiting room to my personal office had eight feet of shelved cupboard space, in two tiers. The top two shelves, which needed to be reached with a step stool, stored drug and dressing supplies. The remaining shelves held office, secretarial, and bookkeeping supplies.

At that point, the bathroom required no revisions, although the shower stall was not used except for storage of supplies. Doors were located at both ends of this corridor between the waiting room and my private office, through which we ushered patients to the main treatment room or to the auxiliary treatment room under the drug shelves.

While Virginia was my first paid employee, Marian, my partner in marriage, was also my unpaid business partner, even before the start of my practice. It wasn't until our children were grown that she became a paid employee. She retired in the spring of 1982, a year before my practice, known as the Jackson Medical Service Corporation, merged with the General Clinic of West Bend. As an unpaid helpmate, Marian still took messages from patients who called me at home in the declining years of my practice.

I have been truly blessed over the years with loyal employees, friends and colleagues. I think our practice was unique in the personal rapport that developed between members of the staff and our patients. I am hopeful that I don't overlook any of them as I give thanks to all.

It might be mentioned here that the solo practice of medicine is much more difficult to embark on now then when I started. In 1983, when we joined the General Clinic, it was obvious that even the three-physician practice I had developed, with ancillary, part-time physicians, would not long survive the ever-increasing burden of paperwork and added costs imposed by Medicare, Medicaid and the insurance bureaucracies. Just recently, we have seen much larger clinics than the General Clinic, of which I am now a part, swallowed up by mega-clinics. Such large clinics have the economic resources enabling them to, at least for the time being, absorb the ever-increasing costs of doing business.

In this dog-eat-dog world, the easy-going relationship between patient and physician, so treasured in memory, is rapidly becoming a thing of the past. I think few of my readers will disagree with my observation that it is unlikely physicians entering medicine now and in the future, or the people they are privileged to serve, will have the same mutually satisfactory relationships as those I have enjoyed.

The pace of life in all areas has so speeded up that it seems "the faster we run, the behinder we get." The practice of medicine has changed as much, or more, than the change in agriculture from the family farms of my youth to the corporate farms of today. The technological advances over the last half century have certainly extended the human life span; but whether the quality of life found in those added years justifies the costs to the individual and society is a moot question. While many of us continue to be productive and enjoy life to the fullest beyond the proverbial three score and ten, most of us in society would probably be better off dying of "the old man's friend," pneumonia, than have our lives extended at a cost of two to three thousand dollars a month to survive — but not really live — in nursing homes, which are destined to eat up an ever-increasing portion of health-care dollars.

Many years ago, Reverend Louis Riesch, whose family I had cared for, started the Cedar Lake Home in Washington County, now one of the outstanding establishments of its kind in the country. In the early years, during one of our discussions, I raised the question as to how long society could afford to keep people in "holding tanks" while awaiting death to return them to

120

their Maker. That question raised over thirty years ago is still faced by society today.

I have long felt that the dream of so many, to be able to retire at age sixty-five, would be a nightmare for me. I daily thank God that He has blessed me with the ability and opportunity to continue practicing my calling, even into my dotage.

16

"Building Friendships"

Within just a few weeks of starting my practice in 1948, it became apparent that the members of the Jackson Village Board wouldn't have to lay awake nights wondering if they'd have to make good on their guarantee of twenty-five hundred dollars the first year. Although money was tight — cash across the counter seldom exceeded five hundred dollars a month and the bills for drugs and equipment ran about six hundred dollars a month — the accounts receivable kept growing.

With largely a farm background, I was aware of the cyclic nature of farmers' income, and their inherent honesty, I told my patients to pay when they could.

The local banker was more realistic and insisted I put up my meager life insurance as collateral on loans I took out to get us through the first year. If more people with this cautious attitude had remained in the banking business, the savings and loan crisis of today would not have occurred!

While I didn't question Elmo Rosenheimer's need to protect his stockholders, he remained my banker for only a year or two before I transferred my accounts to the First State Bank in West Bend, where Mel Gumm's brother, Walter, was an officer. Walter, and his two banking colleagues, remained friends of mine until their deaths.

The First State Bank became part of the Marine Bank system, and in the last few years became part of Bank One. Their officers and employees have remained good friends, over many years.

They weren't the only bankers who befriended me in my lifetime. During my boyhood, Christmas and birthday gifts were put into a savings account at the "Old National Bank" in Beaver Dam, now part of the Valley Bank system. I have fond memories of my personal relationship with various bank presidents and members of the boards of directors to whom I delivered eggs and farm produce during an earlier chapter of my life. They also cooperated with me in some other ventures I'll describe later.

Mr. Chandler, Mr. Fisher and Howard Schoenwetter, all of whom have gone to meet our Maker, and Tom Fisher, the most recent president before the merger with Valley Bank, have a special place in my heart. Tom and Howard arranged a new house mortgage for me during the time of great stress in 1976 when I was named in what I still consider an unjust malpractice suit. I wanted to be certain that none of the people who had lent me money would be left "holding the bag" in the event I lost the suit. I put everything together in one mortgage and got everybody paid off prior to going to court. (The case was later settled out of court.)

I think, as we go through the chronology of my life, it will be apparent to all that when I tell people, "I know how you feel," when they express anxiety and doubts, that in most cases I have experienced the same human reaction to stress.

Somewhat earlier, two other friends, Lee Pinkham and Phil Dressler, officers of M&I Bank in Milwaukee entered the picture after I had read an article in *Medical Economics* about the Clifford Trust, which would enable people to provide for the education of their children. I realized that I probably would never save enough for the education of Lynn, Peter and Chuck, our third child. We investigated the feasibility of putting the office building into a Clifford Trust. By that time, the office building had been renovated and expanded several times. (Between 1951, when we bought it from Les Klumb, to 1984 when we sold it to James and Nancy Schultz for its present function as Tri-Manor, a community-based residential facility, we had remodeled a total of nineteen times.)

The concept of the trust was then so new that M&I officers were not yet comfortable with doing this. My old friends at Beaver Dam handled the first ten years of the Albrecht Children Life Insurance and Education Trust. The following ten years, M&I assumed the responsibility. With this mechanism I was forced to pay rent on the property as we went along, and the children obtained their education without the horrendous debt burdening many of the graduates of today as they enter the business of life.

I would be remiss if I didn't mention the necessity of having friends among the legal profession.

Art Spence, long since deceased, had been a member of the Milwaukee Board of Education, and was one of the original teachers of the Dale Carnegie Course in Milwaukee. In 1953, Marian and I realized that all work and no play made Jim a dull boy and Marian a frustrated wife and mother. We made arrangements with Dr. Frankow and Dr. Grundahl to cover my practice one night a week and signed up for the Dale Carnegie course taught by Art Spence. Sometimes we would have time to go into Milwaukee and have dinner before the seven o'clock start of the class. Sometimes we would barely get there because of delays in finishing office hours. But, at least for ten weeks, we did have a weekly date.

By rubbing shoulders with people of various professions and jobs of varying economic strata, we developed a greater understanding and empathy for others of different backgrounds. I am not sure if either Art Spence or Dale Carnegie (We did have the good fortune of having him attend our graduation.) would be happy to acknowledge that I not only graduated from the first course, but took the advanced course led by Art Spence.

Among other things, Art impressed on us the value of having a will, even at a young age, as well as having a common sense approach to various things in life. Art suggested that I start out by having him draw up a will and that was accomplished. It was only natural when I heard about the Clifford Trust to ask him to investigate and later to get the "show on the road." He and his young colleagues arranged for the purchase of the three acres on which our home now stands, or at least arranged for the legal niceties in 1955. My friends at Beaver Dam arranged for the mortgage on the home we moved into in 1956 and in which we still reside. That mortgage had been paid off by the time of our silver wedding anniversary in 1969, current encumbrance as noted.

In the course of my practice, I occasionally became involved in testifying in court and have developed friendly relations with many of the lawyers and all of the judges in Washington County.

Having been county coroner from 1952 to 1959, I have had a good relationship with members of the Sheriff's Department, as well as with members of the legal profession, and a continuing cordial relationship with my medical colleagues.

I noted that the Schloemer Law Office in West Bend had a

disproportionate number of former members as judges. Clyde Schloemer and his wife Myrtle had started out his practice of law in somewhat the same manner Marian and I had started out in the practice of medicine. He too had been a farm boy, and we developed an empathy which is necessary if you are to have blind trust in your advisors.

When Art Spence died, I called Clyde. I told him that, while I had no pressing legal problems I knew of, I would appreciate visiting with him to see if we could establish the same mutually satisfying relationship Marian and I had enjoyed with Art Spence. Clyde and his wife accepted our invitation to dinner at our home, and we learned how closely our struggles of youth corresponded.

The evening with Clyde and Myrtle was pleasant and our relationship over the years, until their deaths, was a friendly one. Clyde suggested that it would be well for him to go over our wills again and thus establish an attorney-client relationship. Our mutually satisfying friendship continued with his assigning various younger people in his office to do specific tasks for me in their area of expertise.

Later, as he got older, Clyde arranged for my present personal attorney, Jim Spella, to succeed him some years before Clyde died. I think it is as important for people to establish a relationship with an attorney as it is important for patients to establish a rapport with a personal family physician.

Clyde and his wife established their practice during the time I was farming and returning to high school. His uncle, Adolph Schloemer, had been the physician in Jackson just preceding my predecessor, Dr. Froede.

Dr. Schloemer, who was then in his sixties, still drove to Jackson to make home calls for the same four dollar charge I had established, although he didn't charge mileage. I charged seventy-five cents a mile. We were friendly competitors.

I recall some years later pronouncing him dead, after he had

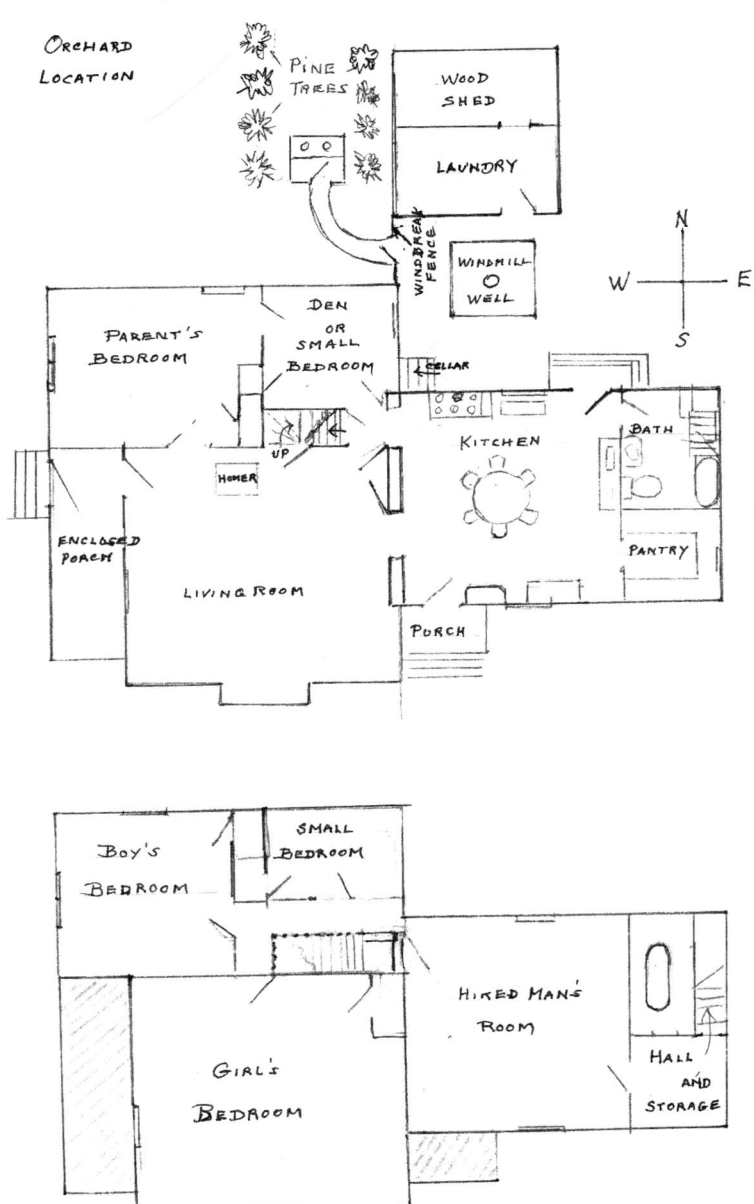

Orchard
Location

Pine
Trees

Wood
Shed

Laundry

Windbreak
Fence

Windmill
Well

N

W E

S

Parent's
Bedroom

Den
or
Small
Bedroom

Cellar

Bath

Kitchen

Homer

Up

Pantry

Enclosed
Porch

Living Room

Porch

Boy's
Bedroom

Small
Bedroom

Hired Man's
Room

Girl's
Bedroom

Hall
and
Storage

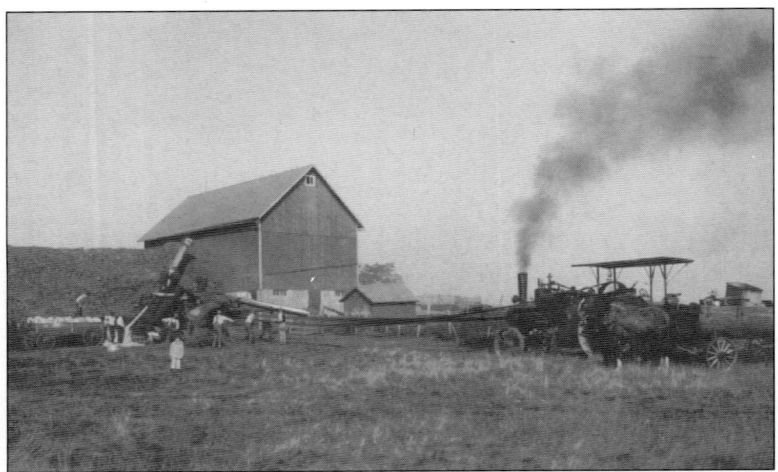

Above: Threshing on Uncle Walde's farm before I was old enough to ride on the water wagon (about 1920).

Right: Grandpa and Grandma Albrecht with Mother and Dad, me, Marjorie, and Harry at the capitol in Madison.

Bottom: Family picture six years before my arrival.

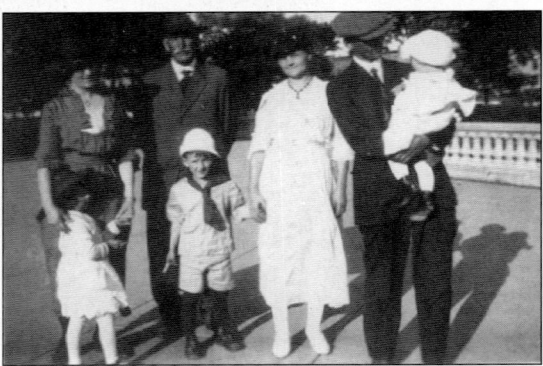

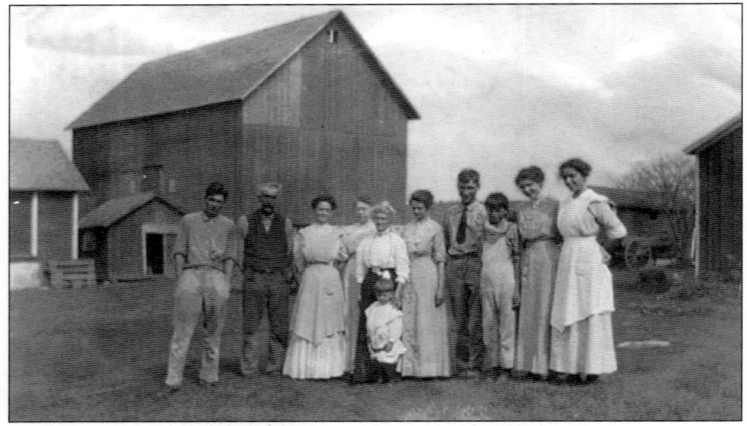

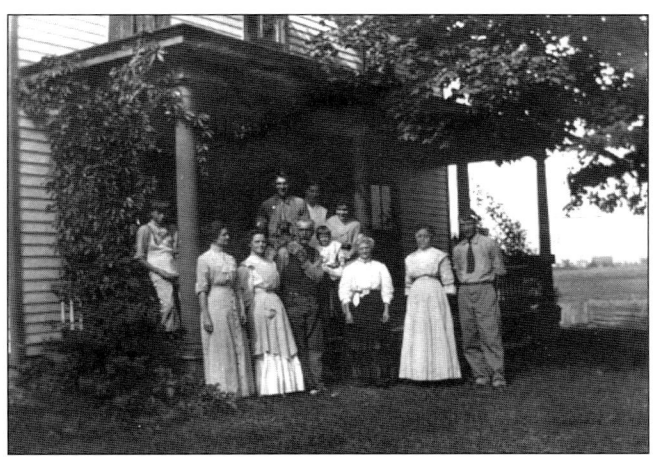

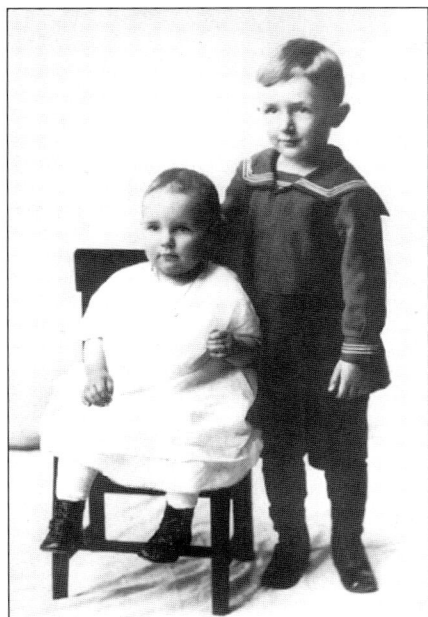

Above: Grandpa Albrecht's house. Family gathering of the past largely unknown today.

Left: With my sister, Marjorie.

Bottom: With Marjorie on south porch off kitchen.

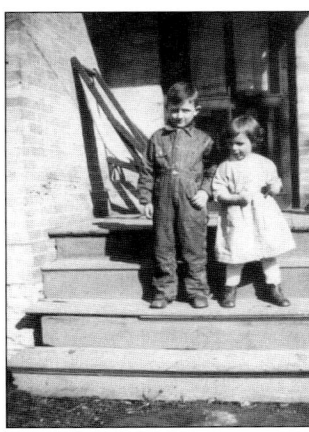

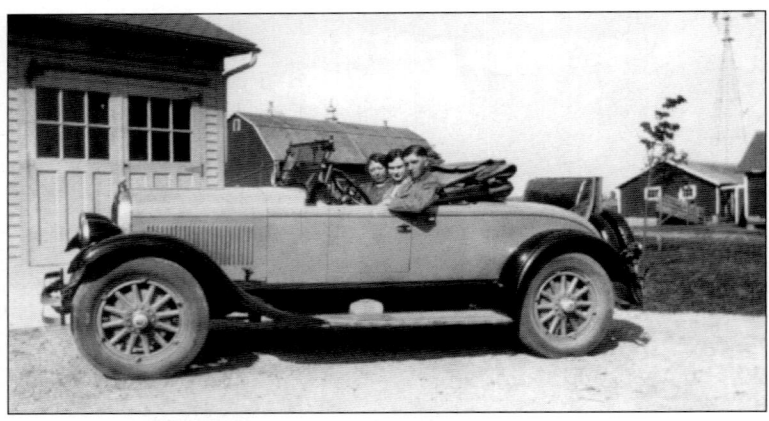

Above: Ervin Miller at Uncle Art Heuer's farm in early 1920s.

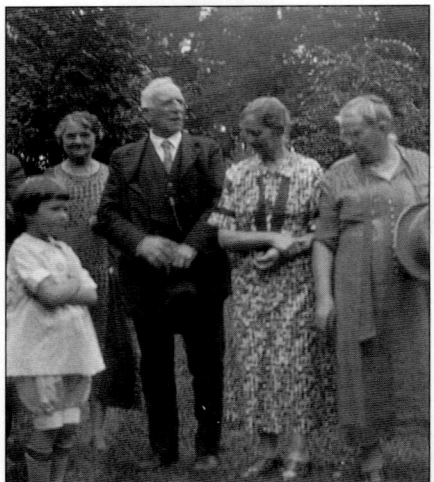

Left: Grandma and Grandpa Keil with Justine Blockwitz, Great Aunt Margaret Pederman and Great Aunt Lizzie Schultz. Swan Park in Beaver Dam in 1926.

Bottom: Unusual tricycle. I'm at the Schaeffer farm, Mayville.

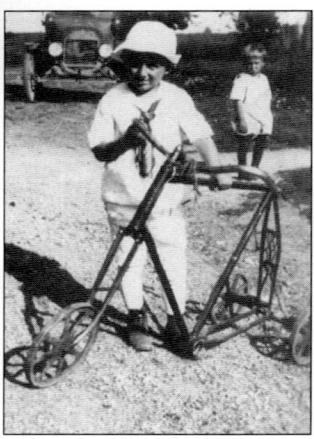

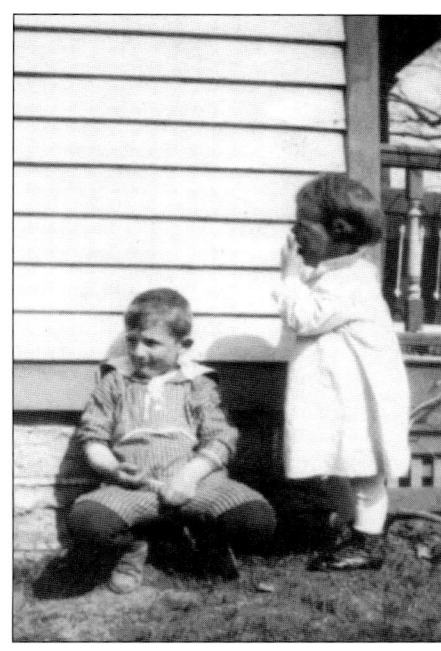

Right: Marjorie and I are at Grandpa Albrecht's house about 1920.

Bottom: Jim Albrecht

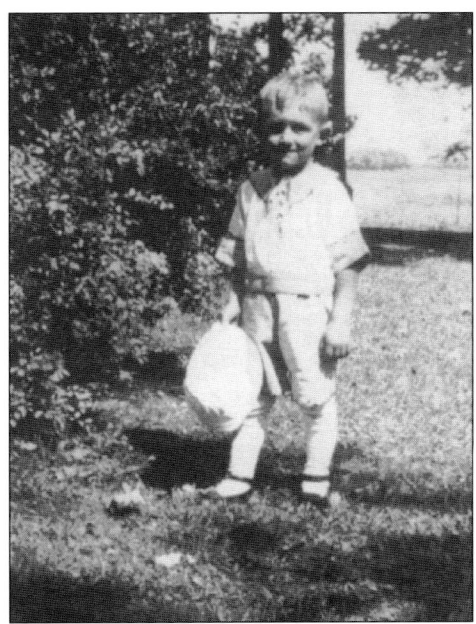

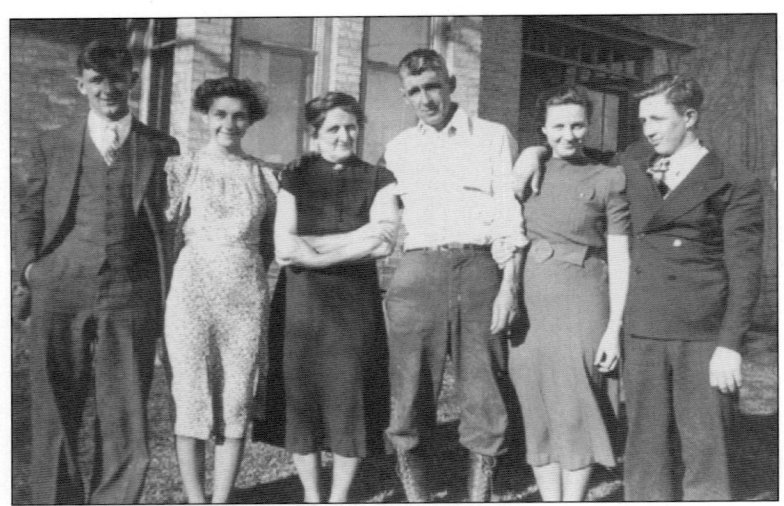

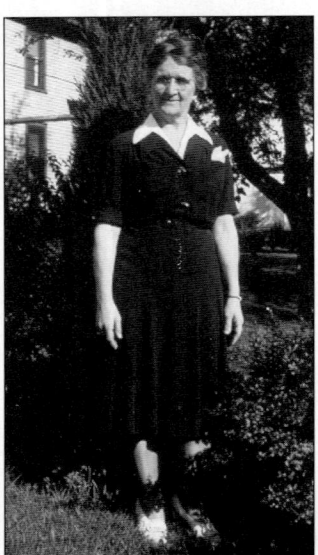

Above: Last picture of the entire family.

Left: Mother as a widow before her second marriage.

Bottom: With my baby sister, Carol.

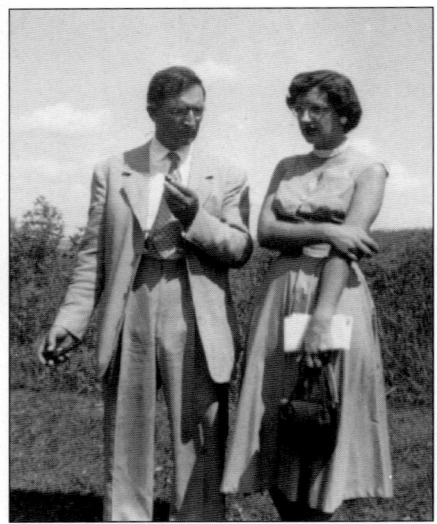

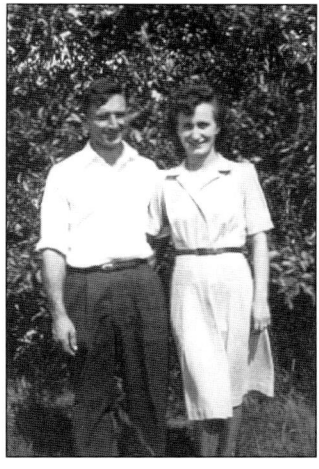

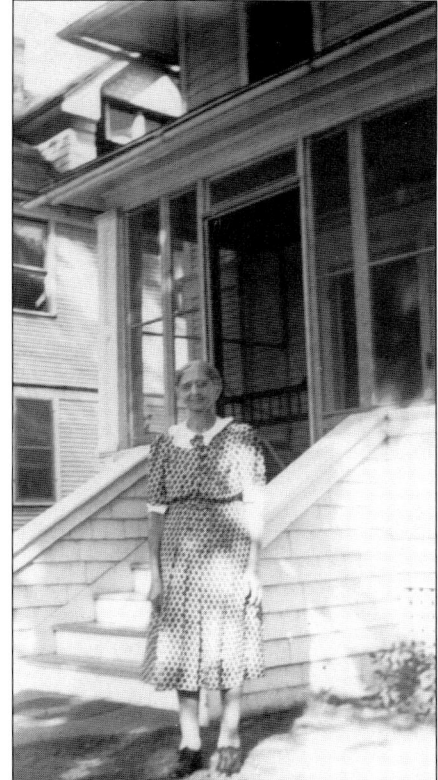

Above: Don't sit under the apple tree with anyone else but me.

Right: Grandma Keil in front of her home.

Bottom: Grandma Albrecht (rear) with Aunt (Roni) Veronica (left); Mother (Cora Albrecht), center; and Aunt Alma Kellorn.

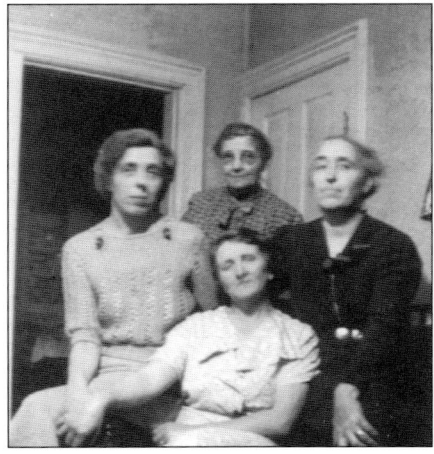

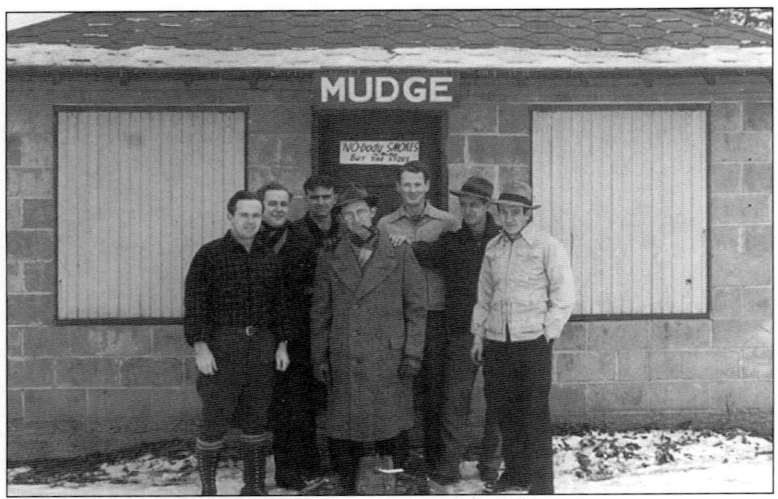

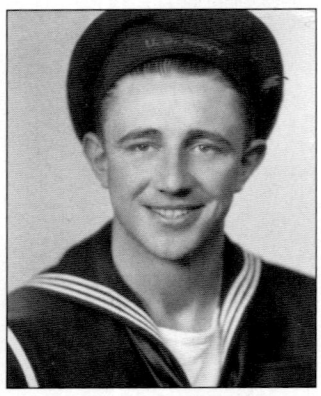

Above : Adieu from Merom CPS Camp 14 enroute to Cleveland State Hospital in 1942.

Left: Brother Harry.

Bottom: Marian's first picture with my family.

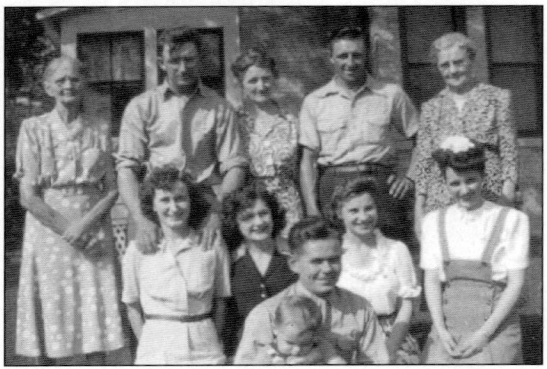

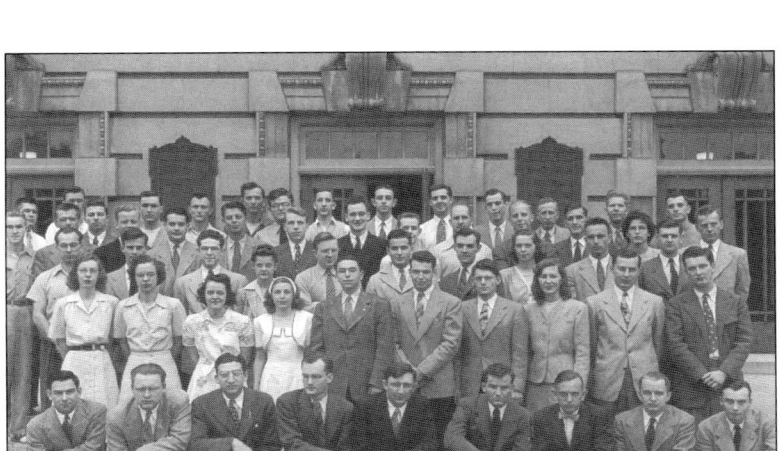

Above: Medical School Class of 1947. I'm in the center of the bottom row.

Right: Dr. James Albrecht, MD and daughter at graduation from medical school in 1947.

Bottom: Campaign poster portrait for Washington County coroner race in 1952.

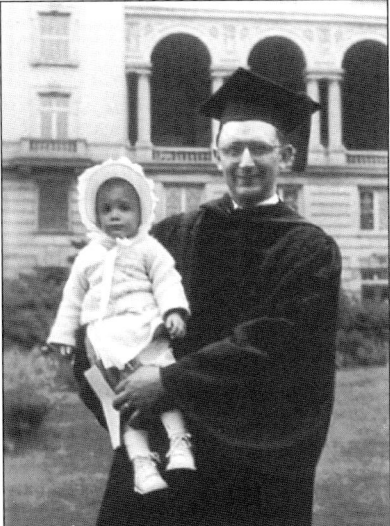

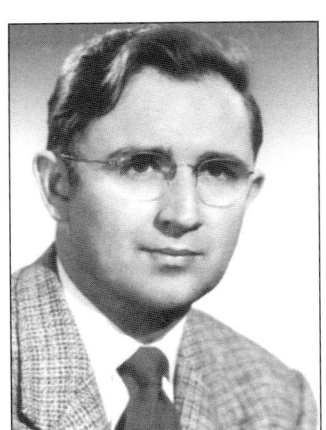

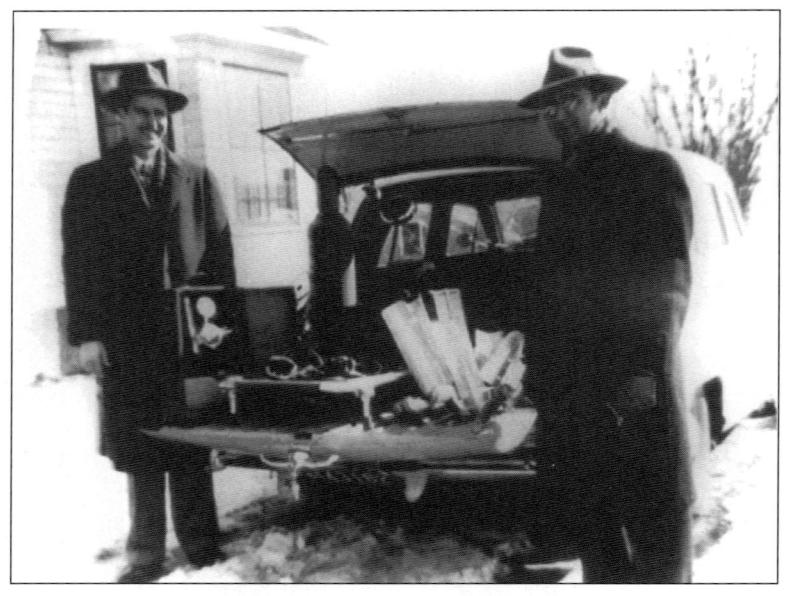

Above: I provided the first ambulance in Washington County. This Kaiser-Fraser was sold and equipped by John Gumm in January, 1949.

Bottom: My early equipment is now a part of history at the Washington County Historical Society.

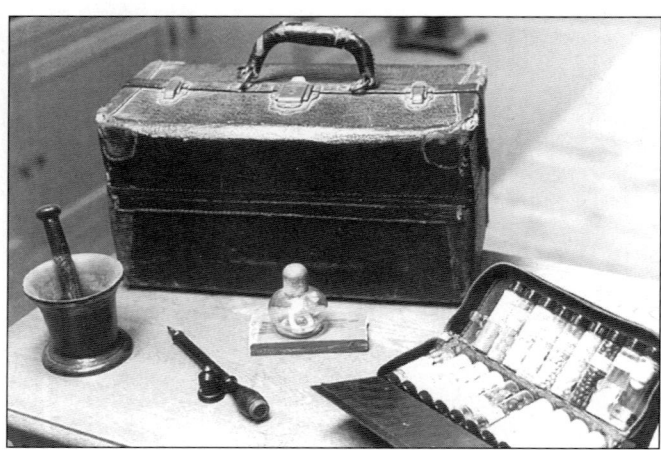

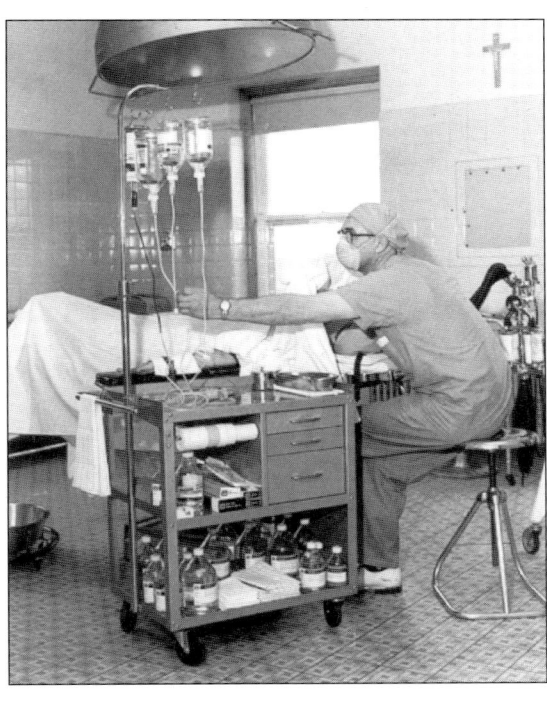

Above: A sideline – designing, manufacturing, and marketing the O.R.A. anesthesia tables.

Left: My first shingle and only daughter.

Bottom: Preceptor and preceptee.

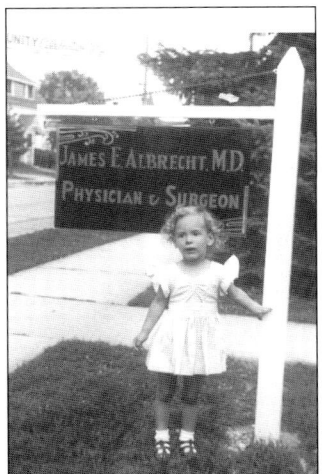

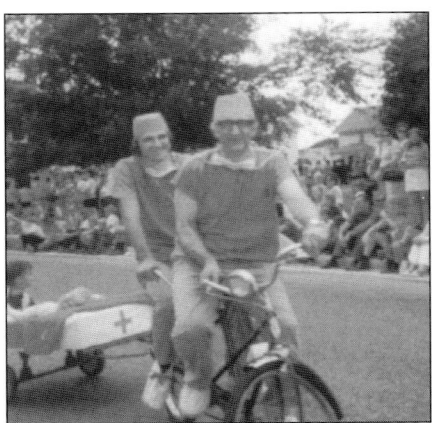

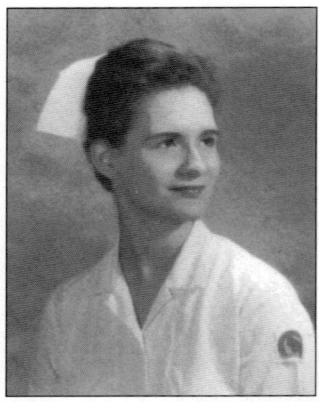

Above: Lynn Albrecht as a graduate LPN in 1965.

Right: Appreciation party when medical students Gary Herdrich and Randy Meyer reciprocated for 10 weeks of intensive training by trying to drown me towing on water skis under the surface of Silver Lake.

Bottom: Three doctors in the family:(Left) Dr. James Albrecht; Dr. Jesse Vegafria, son-in-law; Dr. Charles Albrecht, son.

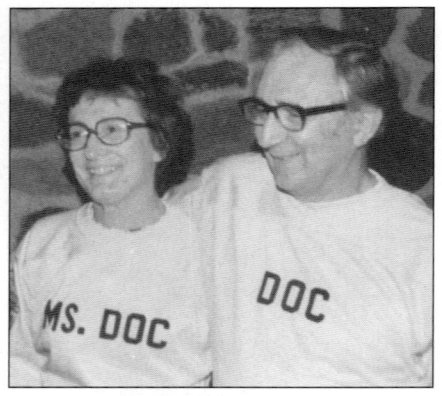

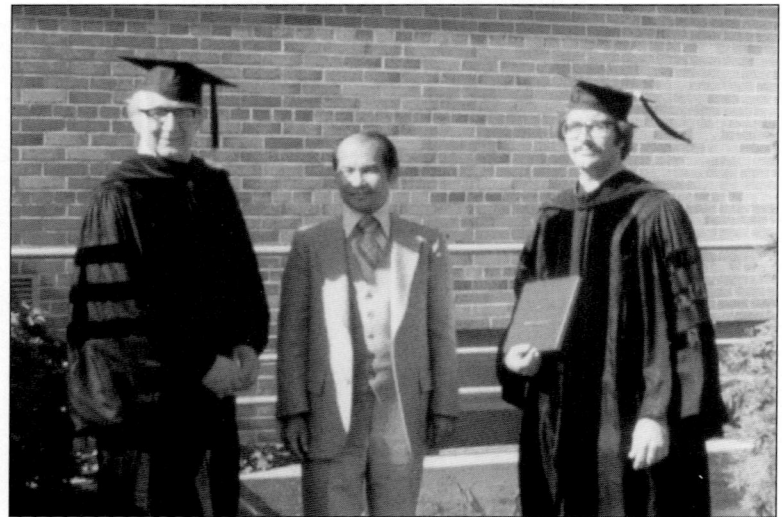

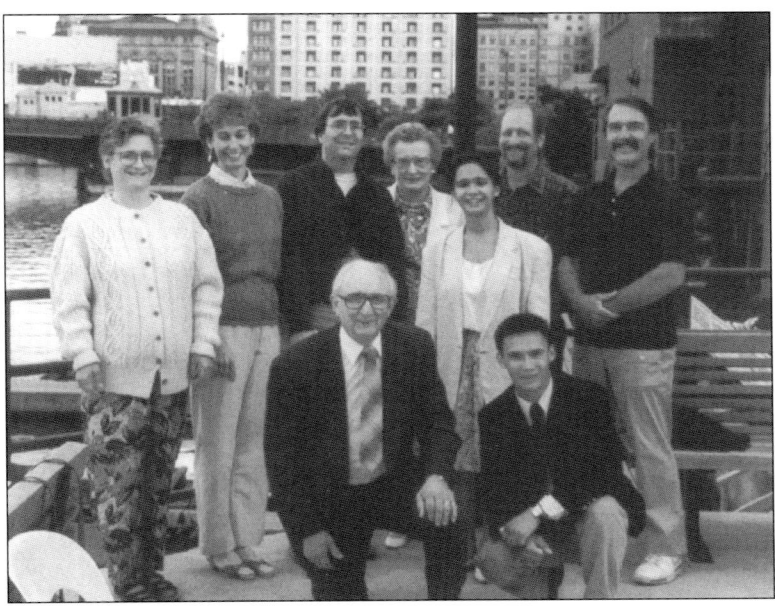

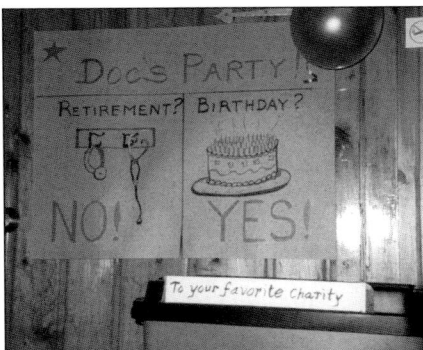

Above: Marian's 70th birthday party with all of the immediate family except for Pete's wife, Becky and, Lynn's husband, Jesse who had to work. Our good friend, Bob Ditlow, joined us.

Above: My 75th birthday party raised thousands of dollars for 35 charities and I provided about 650 pots to my friends. 950 meals were served.

Right: Dancing to the Anniversary Waltz at my 75th birthday party.

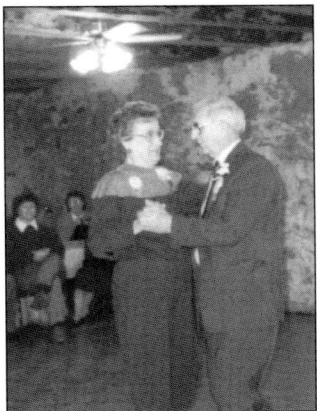

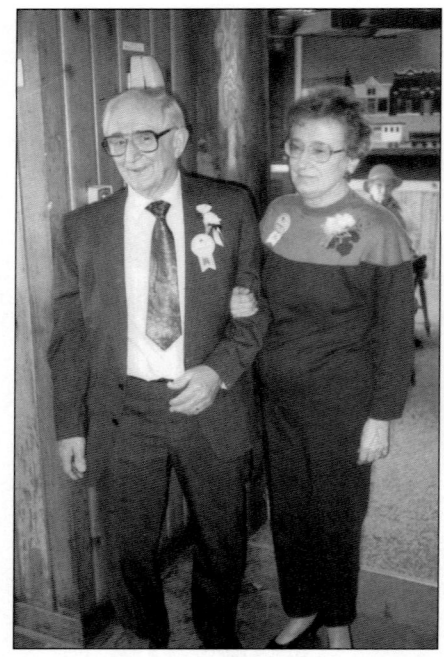

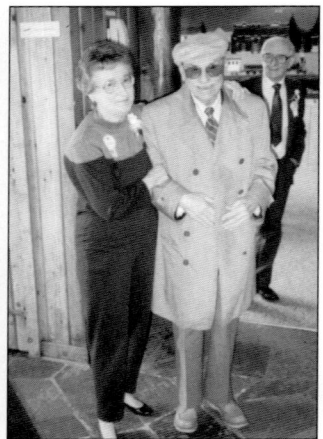

Above: Willard Oehrlein, Marian's relative, came to celebrate my 75th birthday.

Left: On our way to the barn to dance the Anniversary Waltz at my 75th birthday party.

Bottom: Vegafria family: Lynn, Jesse, Cora, and David.

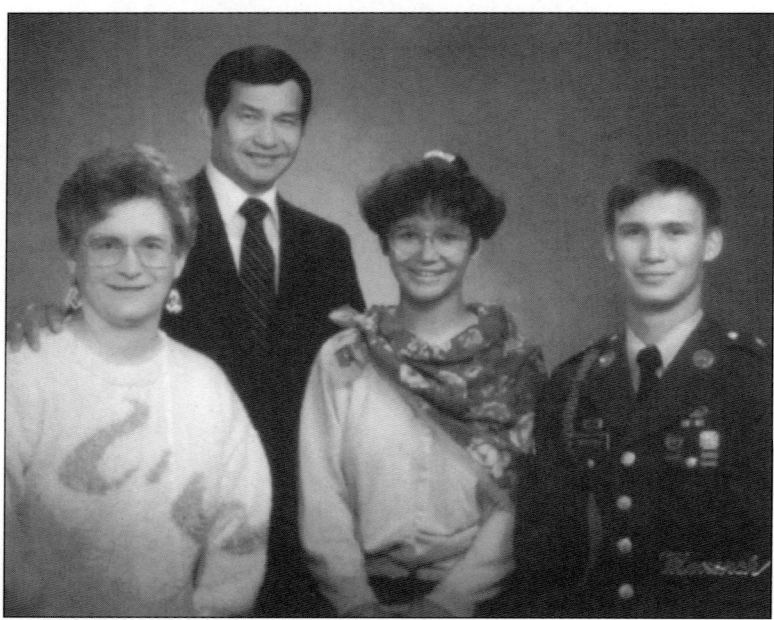

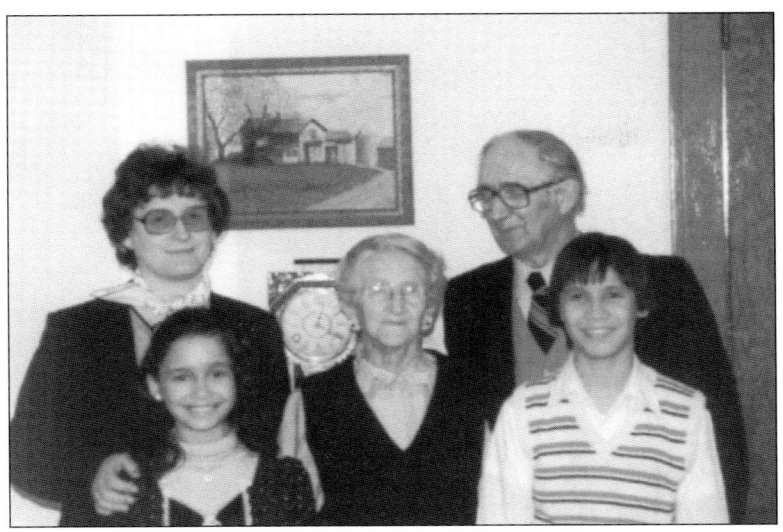

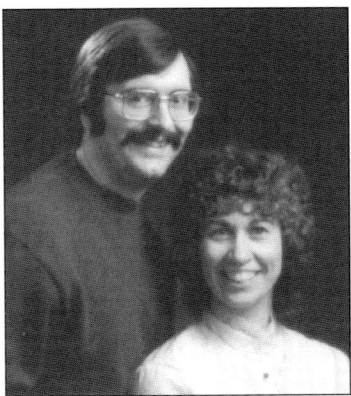

Above: Four generations. My mother, Cora Cain; me; my daughter, Lynn; and grandchildren David and Cora. A picture of the old farmhouse in the background.

Left: Charles Albrecht and Linda Struble.

Bottom: Peter Albrecht and Becky Moody.

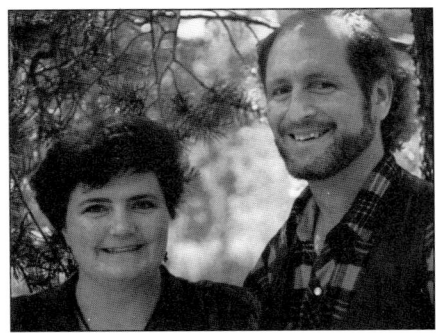

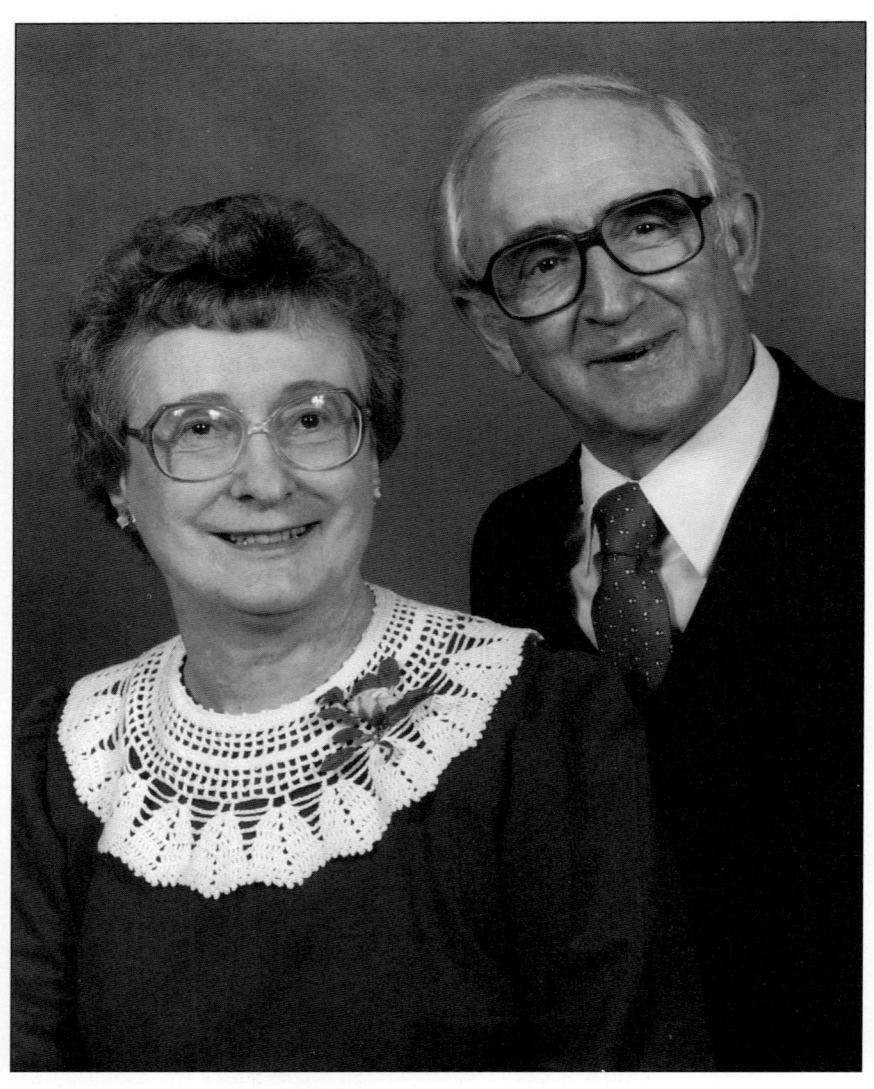

Jim and Marian Albrecht. November, 1987.

a heart attack while driving on one of his patient calls. His car slowly ran off County Highway G near Jackson into a field about one-half mile south of State Highway 60. (At that time Dr. Schloemer, Dr. Dohman, and Dr. Dewerth were the only three active doctors in Menomonee Falls, located about fifteen miles south of Jackson in Waukesha County.)

Dr. Dohman helped my practice develop earlier than I had expected. He called and asked a favor of me. He wanted me to help him preserve his practice by taking night and weekend calls in the Germantown area while his two sons finished medical school and residency.

In this day of the vanishing general practitioner, the ever-increasing fragmentation of medicine with specialty practices, and the growth of the corporate practice of medicine, the personal relationship between patient and physician is becoming largely a matter of fond memory. The necessary attention to the business of medicine makes it unlikely that the young physicians of today will have the same fond memories I am trying to share.

Few will be blessed with the experiences I have enjoyed since 1953 with Professional Management Consultants, founded by Oscar Gaarder and Paul Miller. The founders of the firm visited my home and office by invitation in the spring of 1953 when I was having a dispute with the Wisconsin income tax people.

The dispute was over my drug inventory methods. While I had done an actual count on May 1 each year since 1949 for local tax purposes, I did not do a December 31 drug inventory. At that time, when I was dispensing drugs, most of the drugs were not paid for by the patients until some months later. Sometimes, I sold the drugs to my patients for a ridiculously low mark-up. If I bought ten thousand of a particular pill and I dispensed them in one hundred lots, I divided the total cost per hundred lots and charged the patient that amount without adding anything for the cost of the container or my time. Subsequently, when the pills were paid for (sometimes months or years later), I paid income tax on the total receipts. The tax people insisted that I pay tax on the increase of my drug inventory from year to year as of December 31, and they would not accept my May 1 actual inventory for each year since I started practice.

When state revenue service officials insisted they needed an actual December 31 inventory, I suggested that they might wish to send an auditor to my office to establish what the inventory was at the end of each of the preceding years. This invitation was accepted.

The auditor sat in our dining room with the records, which we had methodically kept, brought to him from the office by one of my employees at his request. When he completed his job on the third day, he wanted me to sign a statement that the figures he had arrived at were my December 31 drug inventories for each of the preceding four years, and that I owed taxes on them. I told him it was impossible for me to sign that without fear of perjury and ended up writing on the form, "This is what Mr. So-and-so says my tax obligation was on each of these years," before I signed and dated it. I wrote a check for some seven hundred-eighty dollars and included the check with the auditor's calculations, taking the precaution of keeping a copy for my records.

I knew it would be only a matter of time until the state revenue service communicated to the federal Internal Revenue Service, so the very next day I called Gaarder and Miller, professional management counselors who had opened their office a few years earlier in Madison. They were already serving many physicians in the western and central areas of Wisconsin when I heard about them and decided to call. Within a few days both Oscar and Paul came to Jackson and agreed to become my professional management counselors. Paul personally came to my office once a month until he retired in 1969. He introduced me to his son, John, who continues to visit me, on a less frequent basis since I merged my practice with the General Clinic in 1983.

That experience with the state revenue service led to a rapid change in the practice of medicine, not only in Jackson but, within a few years, in the entire county. I realized I was actually losing money on the drugs I dispensed. In 1953, two young pharmacists, Jim Niebauer and Carl Kircher, had a small pharmacy in downtown West Bend. Mr. Franzel owned a grocery store and had a small pharmacy in Slinger. I believe there were two pharmacies in Menomonee Falls, one in Hartford and two in the Cedarburg-Grafton area.

Expensive antibiotics had only recently become available. Most physicians were still dispensing drugs, but many had developed the habit of writing prescriptions for the more expensive drugs so they didn't have a bloated drug inventory or a lot of expensive drugs in the hands of patients who would not be paying for them. When I spoke to Jim and Carl about the possibility of establishing a drug store in Jackson, they questioned whether a one-physician office could make it worthwhile. I pointed out that they currently weren't making enough between them for even one of them to survive, the way things were going. The forty to sixty patients I was seeing and giving drugs to each day could provide several times the volume they currently were dispensing, I said.

After some discussion and a few days for reflection, the decision was made that I would extensively remodel my office to accommodate a pharmacy.

Jim and Carl would buy out my drug inventory and I would rent them sufficient room for a prescription pharmacy at fifty dollars a month. If they were not making a profit in six months, I would buy back the drugs, release them from their rental agreement, and we would part friends. If after six months they wanted to continue their association in Jackson, we would rene-gotiate a more equitable rental agreement.

Thus started a long-lasting friendship and mutually reward-ing business relationship. It resulted in Jim and Carl establishing similar business relationships with physicians in West Bend. Jim and Carl continued supplying the Jackson Medical Service with pharmacists until we merged with the General Clinic in 1983. For about nine months after the merger, they continued to rent space in my Jackson Office. Shortly thereafter the old office was sold to Jim and Nancy Schultz who converted the two upper floors into the Tri-Manor Home.

Years earlier, I initially thought of expanding my office building to the north, bringing it closer to the sidewalk. Marian had dreams of having a new home out in the country. She sug-gested that we convert the entire first floor of the office build-ing to offices and pharmacy and convert the second floor to an apartment where we could live for a few years until cir-cumstances enabled us to build a separate home. The space was not quite adequate, so plans were made to add one room above my main treatment room. By taking about fourteen inches from the west side of my laboratory and drug room, which, added to a closet, we were able to get a stairway with one landing up to that open porch. Enclosing this porch to make a "knotty-pine" room gave us five rooms and a bathroom to live in, with added storage space in the attic.

Three smaller, prior remodelings had converted the entire enclosed porch on the front end of the building into a large waiting room. The central of three windows of our living room was converted into a split door with a ledge at chest height so that patients in the waiting room could get their prescribed drugs at that counter. Windows on either side of this were closed. The swinging door over the counter top closed and locked when the office was not open.

The arch between the living and dining rooms was closed

off, with a similar counter space and swinging door connecting the south side of the pharmacy to the little corridor serving three small treatment rooms. These three rooms were formed by partitioning the dining room into two and the south side of the kitchen into one. This provided a corridor with a small treatment room to the south, with the original countertops, cabinets and sink of the old kitchen to the north of the corridor. A doorway was cut through the east wall of the old kitchen to provide a connecting arched entry from the new portion of the office into the old. We thus had six treatment rooms, three in my old office and three in the space which had once been the kitchen and dining room. Our old living room became the pharmacy. The pharmacists had shelves built to their specifications.

The whole house was insulated, windows and stormwindows custom fitted. The stairway and knotty-pine room were built, the bathroom renovated, and one bedroom made into a kitchen with an outside vent for the hood over the stove. A patient and friend, Martin Bauman, planned the conversion, the building inspector expedited the permit, a youthful contractor, patient and friend, Harold (Rusty) Kloehn, accomplished the miracle of getting the job done within thirty days from the concept of the plan until our family moved to the apartment upstairs.

The work was so integrated and carefully planned that we lost only a day and a half of office hours during the conversion. An open house two Sundays after the conversion was completed introduced our patients, friends and the community to our newly remodeled facility and our pharmacist friends.

CHAPTER

17

"Employees and Friends"

M arian had been my helpmate both in life and the practice of medicine from the day of our marriage on August 18, 1944. Not only did she almost single-handedly care for our three children, but until our children were old enough to go to school, as an unpaid business partner, she kept track of where the doctor was, and answered the phone, both day and night, when paid employees were not at the office.

Marian became a paid employee from the time our son Charles started school until her retirement in 1982. We held a surprise retirement party at our home for her, attended by former employees and fellow members of the Sweet Adeline's, with whom she had enjoyed singing for several years. Yet, despite her return to unpaid status for the last ten years, she still continued to answer the phone and tried to keep track of where I was until her death December 7, 1992. (She had edited this chapter a day before her stroke.)

My first paid employee in the practice of medicine was Virginia Gilbert, whose husband, Howard, died at an early age before I came to Jackson. Her mother and two brothers lived in Jackson. Originally, she was employed by Melvin Gumm, owner of the Hoge & Gumm General Store. Since he was one of the village board who had guaranteed me a gross income of twenty-five hundred dollars the first year, he was easily prevailed on to let me ask Virginia to work for me.

I doubt there are many employees today who would offer as Virginia did to help get the house in order after evening office hours the night before Marian was to return home from Milwaukee Hospital, after a ten-day postpartum stay following the birth of our son Peter (born September 27, 1948).

Virginia was a valued employee who was acquainted with the people of Jackson and surrounding area. She continued to work for me even after she married Elroy Borchardt and until I delivered her son in 1953, the same year our Chuck was born.

During Marian's hospitalization, Lynn stayed with Marian's parents in Milwaukee. I was still doing anesthesia at Milwaukee Hospital when Peter was born. Marian's roommate was amazed when an intern in his operating room clothing came in and kissed Marian a few hours after her baby was born!

Prior to hiring Virginia and prior to obtaining my license to practice medicine, we had arranged to provide room and board to an older girl from the Martha Washington Home for Unwed Mothers To Be. I had worked a maternity rotation there as an intern. She was a girl who felt picked on by the other residents at the Martha Washington Home, and wanted a job so badly that I "hired" her to help Marian in our home and in my office.

After a few weeks, we noticed Lynn had head lice — even

on her eyebrows — presumptively acquired from our guest and pseudo-employee. Those in charge at the maternity home were chagrined and apologetic. A year later, after we bought the house in which my office was located, the Martha Washington Home provided us with a personable girl whose parents were happy to have her in a private home. She was not only helpful, but good company. We were sorry she had to leave when she delivered. She kept in contact with us for a year after she left.

As the office workload increased, we needed more help. Clarence and Marvel Kurtz were fellow members of Christ Lutheran Church. Marvel agreed to work for me as a receptionist and bookkeeper so that Virginia could help me care for patients. Marvel worked for me for four or five years and remains a patient and friend.

Early dictation equipment, including tape recorders and a Grey audiograph, to me appeared to be the thing of the future — especially for one whose handwriting was difficult to read. Joyce Rose, a high school student, became a part-time employee transcribing letters and insurance reports. (In those days I dictated all insurance reports, even if it meant being at the office until after midnight.) Joyce worked as a part-time employee until her graduation and as a full-time employee until she married and had children. For several years she again worked for me as a part-time employee, when her household duties permitted. Ultimately, as she was dying of a blood dyscrasia and couldn't get to the office anymore, she still had a typewriter and transcription device in her home so she could continue helping me as her strength permitted.

Joyce was the first of numerous girls who were hired during their junior or senior year of high school. As I recall, this group included Geraldine Junghans, the eldest of eleven children in a financially strapped family belonging to our church. Jerry, her father, was a skillful jack-of-all-trades, who helped me out with office maintenance jobs.

Geraldine dreamed of becoming a nurse. At the time, her dream seemed almost as impossible as my earlier ambition to be a doctor. When I hired her, it was with the agreement she would save half of her earnings for school. After part-time work during her junior and senior years of high school and full-time employment during summer vacation, she asked me if we could modify our agreement to allow her to use the savings as a down payment on the first house her family ever owned. She also asked if I would hire her full-time for another year to replenish her college fund.

Not only did she go on to get her Registered Nurse degree, but she became the wife of a pastor, now retired. She currently teaches at the School of Nursing at University Hospitals in Madison.

Other part-time student helpers over the years included Darlene Faber, Debbie Carson, Cheri Rose, Jan Junghans, Lynn Arnold, Judy Chantelois, Joan Hauser, Kay Johnson and my daughter, Lynn Vegafria.

Lynn also remembers another employee of mine, Rhoda Woodard, RN, working with her during my Friday evening vasectomy hours.

I was an equal opportunity employer. I had one of the first male employees doing office work in a physician's office early in the 1950s. His name was Roy Koehn. Later, in the 1960s, Bernie Hauser, the father of Joan, became a valued employee for a number of years.

Other employees I remember with affection include Vi Miller and her daughter Sonia.

Vi and Sonia probably have the distinction of having volunteered for the most unusual extracurricular activity enjoyed by any physician's assistants. One summer day, as a neighbor farmer baled the hay on our three-acre homestead, rain was forecast. Vi and Sonia volunteered to come out and help me bring the bales from the field into the barn with their pick-up truck, thus saving the hay from getting wet. We used the hay to help feed the sheep herd we raised in our backyard.

In the early 1960s, as our children were growing up, I had the idea that children should have chores to justify their allowances. Since we had three acres, we developed two sizable pastures in an "L" shape around the south and east portion of our home and built a sizable barn with a hayloft. We bought two sheep, Ruth and Naomi, which we had bred when they reached a suitable age. Our children helped care for the sheep.

The initial sheep house was built with the help of my father-in-law and Jerry Junghans, out of mink houses bought at a bargain from some mink ranches going out of business in the Cedarburg area. This early sheep house probably was the only one ever to have stained glass windows we also bought for a bargain somewhere — which were broken within a few weeks of installation. Looking back, it seems crude of me to sacrifice perfectly good stained glass windows to such an endeavor.

Subsequently, the barn was built a few years later, when our sheep herd had reached a total of twenty-seven.

Jeanette Sixel was my first RN employee. Alice Liesener Stauss, who was our next-door neighbor when we moved to Jackson, was one of three daughters of Alfred and Anita Liesener, all of whom became nurses. Alice is now our church organist. While she no longer works for me, I see her frequently.

I once tried to give up smoking. After several months of what apparently was some rather crotchety abstinence, Sherry Wolf, another RN who worked for me for a few years, handed me a long-forgotten pipe loaded with my favorite tobacco. She had lit it herself, stating that without the tempering affects of the pipe "we can't stand you any more."

Thus, Sherry holds the distinction of calling to my attention that I was no longer a fit person to work with.

The other RN I recall is Jan Schneider, who was with me a few years before I merged my practice with the General Clinic.

Laurie Reseburg Ksioszk, a licensed practical nurse (LPN), started working for me in 1981 and was one of the employees transferred when we joined the General Clinic.

Elaine LaCharite, also a member of my church, worked for us from 1961 to 1979. I recall asking her in church, just before I left for a postgraduate course in St. Louis, if she would consider working for us. If so, I told her, she should call Vi Miller the next day and arrange to get started on my return from St. Louis. She did.

The maintenance people I recall, Jerry Junghans, Alma Kannenberg and LaVerne Woldt, are all deceased. So is Erla Sullivan, who, together with Vi Miller, handled the books, not only of the Jackson Medical Service, Corp., but two ill-fated business ventures, ORA Table Company, Inc., and Rectangle Tool and Die.

Marianne Ziemann, my lab technician for many years prior to our joining the General Clinic, continued her employment with the General Clinic after the merger. Julie Rehm, another of my former employees, worked with Marianne for several years in Jackson.

Catherine Johnson, mother of Kay, had worked for me many years prior to joining the General Clinic. Until two years ago, when she retired, Catherine continued to work for the General Clinic. She still comes in every six or eight weeks to cut my hair.

Mary Stoiber, who handled the bookkeeping machine for many years, did not follow us to the General Clinic. Sue Cessop-Calhoun, a valued employee for many years, out of friendship still visits my home periodically to get my books ready for John Miller to go over, keeping me out of trouble. She also takes care of the books for Marian's and my business partnership, Painter and Potter.

My current assistant, Dolores Mayer, has worked with me now for twenty-five years.

I think Debbie Racette was the last person I hired a year or so before we joined the General Clinic. She was hired as a record librarian. Other former employees are Chris Scholz and Jane Menke, both of whom handled insurance work over some years.

In the early years of my practice, Dr. Wallace Scheuneman, then a ophthalmology resident and now retired, and Dr. John Palese shared time on weekends so I could get away. Dr. Harry Evans was with me for a little over a year and a half, from 1953 to 1955, before he left for an anesthesiology residency. Dr. James Schultz was with me for about a year and a half in the early '60s and then again for a few months before his death in the early '70s.

My son-in-law, Dr. Jesse Vegafria, practiced family medicine and anesthesiology. He stayed with me from 1969 until 1982, when he limited his practice to anesthesiology.

Dr. Bruce Griswold and Dr. Larry Gill each worked for me one afternoon a week and took calls that same night under a special arrangement with the Frankow-Gundahl Clinic. That enabled me to get started again with my hobby of "throwing pots."

Time share arrangements with physicians from the Parkview Clinic and Hartford Clinic during the '70s and early '80s, as well as with Dr. Muhammad (Joe) Khan enabled us to carry on until the arrival of Dr. Sandra Byerly and Dr. Gary Herdrich, fresh out of residency at Milwaukee's St. Michael's Hospital, in July, 1981.

I think it is notable that, except for Dr. Evans who was contacted through an ad in the *Wisconsin State Medical Journal*, and Debbie Racette who was contacted by a telephone call to

Moraine Park Technical Institute for help in locating a candidate for record librarian, that all of the people mentioned in this chapter came to my employ through personal contact.

18

"Social Changes
and
Social Problems"

Small towns such as Jackson have changed as dramatically in the last forty-five years as has the practice of medicine and the occupation of farming. In many respects, then and now are almost as dissimilar as night and day. For several years after our arrival in Jackson, Mr. Joeckel, who had a farm on the western outskirts of the village, ran errands in town with his horse and buggy. The Kruepke farm was only three doors away from our flat, and their cows were pastured just to the north of our home. The calves were sent to market while Marian was nursing Peter, and the bawling of the bereaved mothers made her feel very sad. Now that whole area is built up with homes and light industry.

The changes in social attitudes are even more striking. Rather than a simple trust in one another, there is now cynical distrust in a dog-eat-dog world where everyone looks after himself and the devil takes the hindmost. The neighborliness of the '40s, '50s, and '60s has been replaced by a troubling question: "Who is my neighbor?"

Human nature hasn't changed much since those days. There were greed, illegitimate pregnancies, venereal disease, and sexual exploitation, not much different from the time my father told Harry and me the facts of life. The ever-increasing permissiveness of social customs with sexually explicit movies, television shows, and books make it much more difficult now for children to develop a sense of values. *Lady Chatterley's Lover*, written in 1920 by D.H. Lawrence, was considered very daring then; it is rather tame by comparison with books written today.

During the 1950s there was a growing number of illegitimate pregnancies and occasional cases of gonorrhea. There was an appalling lack of understanding of human sexuality. Churches in Cedarburg and nearby Slinger, and later the pastor of my own church, invited me to discuss sexuality with their youth groups. We developed a system of speaking to parents and children at the same time, with the groups being broken up for question and answer sessions after the general discussion.

Some of the people in my own church who at first opposed the idea of bringing such a delicate subject into the church, later regretted their opposition when their own children had unwanted pregnancies as a result of ignorance.

In the early 1950s physicians seemed more civic minded than today and regarded free service to our community as a professional obligation. We volunteered to work with the county nurse in putting on immunizations clinics at the different schools, including polio vaccinations when the Salk vaccine became available.

Even in those days, the Washington County Welfare Department found that certain physicians seemed to be overcharging for services rendered to welfare clients. Thus, some of us became involved in monthly meetings to review the charges our colleagues had made and privately remonstrated with those whose charges seemed out of line. Sometimes it seems that the solutions of an earlier day might still be considered as a possible solution to today's rising cost of medical care.

There were three taverns in town. Even though they were responsibly run by law-abiding citizens, those taverns by their very nature contributed to the problem of alcoholism in our society.

In 1953 I needed to commit my uncle Walde to Winnebago State Hospital for treatment of alcoholism. Shortly thereafter, I heard Rev. Lawrence Parish, the head of the United Temperance Movement of Wisconsin, speak at my wife's home church, Bethel Evangelical, in Bay View. His comparison of the disease of alcoholism to infectious diseases, with the germ being alcohol itself, forced me to realize that working with alcoholism was one of the things God would have me do. For seven years I worked with alcoholics in my practice before helping form one of the first chapters of Alcoholics Anonymous in Washington County in 1960.

Ten years later, I felt impelled by the forces of circumstance to help start a drug information council, as a result of the prodding of a Vietnam War veteran. This son of a lab technician at the West Bend hospital raised the question, "Why doesn't Dr. Albrecht, or someone like him, help the young people with drug problems like he has helped the alcoholic?"

Society is now supporting both programs which started out as volunteer efforts in answer to the twin questions, "Who is my neighbor?" and "What would God have me to do?" The problems of alcoholism, drug abuse, and teenage sexual activity have grown greatly since that time. The sexual revolution has resulted in children having children, a phenomenal increase in venereal disease, as well as AIDS. All these result from permissiveness and the loss not only of social control but self control. This lack of responsibility is more likely to destroy our society than cancers and infectious diseases combined.

19

"Emergency Medicine"

On a cold, wet day toward the end of January 1949, a call came about an accident on State Highway 145, a few miles south of Jackson. A young man from Illinois had lost control of his car, crossed the road and forcibly scored a direct hit on the end of a concrete bridge railing.

At that time there were no rescue squads nor ambulances in Washington County. Local undertakers provided injured and ill patients with transportation to the hospital in their "black hacks," which also served to convey the dead. A vehicle from the Schmidt Funeral Home in West Bend had taken one of the women victims of the crash to St. Joseph's Community Hospital. The "ambulance" from Matenaer Funeral Home in Hartford had conveyed the other woman passenger to the Hartford hospital.

The man behind the wheel was thought to be dead. As the closest doctor, I was called to certify him as such and to determine the cause of death.

When I arrived I discovered that, although he had a crushed chest, he was still alive. Passers-by who had stopped to help, opened the trunk of my Chevy sedan, laid my two army blankets on the shoulder of the road and brought my oxygen unit from the trunk. Other people helped me get the man from the car and lay him on the blankets. The oxygen, delivered by mask through a nasal airway, improved his color and circulation so that by the time the hearse from West Bend returned to pick up the "body," the trip was to the hospital rather than to the morgue. The man survived.

At that time, none of the undertakers, fire departments or county officials were willing to provide the ambulance service I perceived as essential. So I decided to do so.

Johnny Gumm had the Kaiser-Fraiser Dealership and Garage at Gumm's Corners at the junction of Sherman Road and State Highway 145. Johnny didn't have a station wagon on his lot and didn't have size measurements of one either. He knew there would be station wagons on display at the annual auto show at State Fair Park in West Allis, a suburb of Milwaukee, held later that week.

We went down to the auto show, carrying a yardstick to measure the station wagons of all the car makers to see which would provide enough room for a stretcher. The Kaiser-Fraiser station wagon was the only one that met our requirements.

A few months earlier, we had flown east on Capital Airlines to visit Marian's brother and his family. On the plane we noticed a folding stretcher, and the stewardess obligingly showed me how it worked when an emergency required it. The aluminum frame made it very light to handle. There were appropriate straps to be placed across the legs and chest of the person to be conveyed out of the airplane and down the steps.

It had folding wheels at one end and legs at the other. This stretcher, I thought, was just what the doctor ordered!

Johnny Gumm was able to procure not only the Kaiser station wagon but the desired stretcher for me in less than two weeks. The station wagon was long enough to comfortably accommodate the six-foot stretcher, leaving a little room to spare for the occasional person over six feet. There was enough space between the back of the front seat and the folded down rear seat to enable John to install a receptacle securely to the floor to safely hold a cylinder of oxygen just behind the passenger side of the car. For the next six years, this ambulance — and its two or three similarly-equipped successor vehicles — was the main emergency vehicle in our area. Not only was I called for medical emergencies, but I also conveyed many accident victims to the hospital.

In the June 1991 issue of *Washington County Health* magazine, free-lance writer Tish Robinson described me as a "country doctor with a mission."

In her article, she quoted the first specialist in West Bend, Dr. C.S. Geiger, an internist who started with the General Clinic in 1969. Dr. Geiger grew up in West Bend. He recalled an incident I had long since forgotten. He "personally remembers Dr. Albrecht's humanitarian efforts in aiding accident victims during the early 1950s."

"My mother was in a severe automobile accident, and although Dr. Albrecht was not her regular physician, he left his office to assist at the scene," Dr. Geiger recounted for the article. "Dr. Albrecht extricated her from the car and did a lot of special things that the Geiger family has always remembered. He was an important ingredient to a good outcome at the time."

It wasn't until 1954 or 1955 that Leander Schmidt of the Schmidt Funeral Home in West Bend and his sons accepted my invitation to take that portion of my business away from me. At about the same time, one of the funeral homes in Menomonee

Falls started transporting the ill and injured in a special vehicle.

About this time, the West Bend and Kewaskum Fire Departments requested I provide some training for their developing rescue squad personnel. Just a few years ago, Brian Mayer, West Bend's fire chief, told me how he found the old McGill forceps I had given the West Bend firemen to use to recover foreign objects from the gullets of choking people.

My availability to work with sheriff's deputies made it natural for me to be made a deputy sheriff so I could have a siren and red lights on my ambulance. During the time the north-south, four-lane U.S. Highway 41 was constructed west of Jackson, I was very busy.

One accident I most clearly remember was a man from Richfield, a township in the south of the county, who fell from one of the highway bridges under construction. He appeared to have fractured ribs and remained conscious for a few hours. After we got him to the hospital, we were troubled by his physical signs of impending doom without any apparent cause.

General practitioner colleagues were the only help available locally. (It wasn't until 1969 that Dr. Charles Geiger became our first resident internal medicine specialist.)

Despite our best efforts, the patient quietly died. His wife graciously gave us permission to do an autopsy. The autopsy was needed so that the coroner could determine cause of death. Performing the autopsy was also important to increase the knowledge of the young doctor in charge and his colleagues.

Even if a specialist had been available, state-of-the-art medicine of the day would have been unlikely to have achieved a much better outcome than we had. Although a chest surgeon may have been able to aspirate the blood that filled the pericardial sac around the man's heart, which caused the ever decreasing pulse we noted clinically, it is unlikely the ruptured auricular appendage could have been fixed. Now, forty years later, such a patient would be whisked off by a Flight For Life helicopter to either Froedtert Hospital or one of the other Milwaukee hospitals for surgery, and would probably survive.

The use of my ambulance was a service I provided in a caring way, with no more financial remuneration than I received dispensing drugs. Patients were charged my usual professional fee for the time involved and seventy-five cents per mile, the same as a home call.

The ambulance was my professional vehicle, with an added bonus. For some years, members of my staff rode with me in the annual Action In Jackson parade.

At that time, it was thought that carbon tetrachloride fire extinguishers should be installed in strategic places in homes and offices. Not only did I provide my home and office with the then state-of-the-art fire prevention, I had one installed under the hood of each of my vehicles. About 2:30 one morning, I had returned home from the hospital after delivering twins for a farmer living three or four miles away. I was just taking off my shoes, looking out our south bedroom window when I saw a glow in the sky coming from that farmer's home. Marian told the local operator to call the Fire Department.

Not yet having gotten completely undressed, I dressed faster than the firefighters and proceeded in my ambulance to the Oliver Vogel residence.

Oliver had not yet gotten home from the hospital and the door to the kitchen was unlocked. I opened the hood of my ambulance and took out my carbon tetrachloride extinguisher. Pulling the stove pipe from the chimney, I aimed my extinguisher at the flames. The fire was extinguished — and I was almost extinguished!

The plastic frames of my glasses melted and my heart was beating rapidly (in excess of 180 per minute). Just as I staggered toward the door, two firefighters met me and escorted me outside. One said, "Doc, you don't look good."

I protested I would be okay as soon as I got my other glasses and they let me drive home. By that time my pulse rate was down to 140 and I was feeling quite a bit better. Even so, I thought I better call one of my internal medical consultants in Milwaukee, Dr. Cy Evans. As he sleepily answered the phone, I told him my symptoms. He suggested that since I was getting better, I would probably totally recover. He said I should call him at seven and let him know how I was doing.

Except for needing to get new glasses, I quickly recovered.

20

"A Few
Emergency Calls,
1949–1955"

The tale recalled when Muriel Kroening sent a postcard that became the impetus for this book is one of the few in which I intended to use the actual names of people involved. In October 1992, Marian and I went to Jimmy's restaurant in Jackson after church and were pleasantly surprised to have a chance to visit with Carl and Laura Seidenstecker. They were sharing a family dinner with some of their children and grandchildren. When I told them that my experience with their family was a catalyst for my autobiography, they graciously gave me permission to use their names.

Even forty years ago, three generations sharing a home was not common. Today it is almost unheard of. The Seidensteckers' large farm home accommodated the older generation in an upstairs flat, while Carl and Laura and their children lived on the lower level. All three generations shared the basement and attic.

I had attended Grandma and Grandpa Seidenstecker on home calls for various reasons a few months prior to an emergency call from Carl and Laura that occurred just at the close of office hours one stormy winter evening. Their two-and-a-half-year-old Ellen had fallen into a pail of scalding water in the barn. They had been mixing hot water with cold to wash cows' udders prior to applying the milking machine.

When they called, the family had already taken off Ellen's snow suit. I instructed them to wrap her in a clean sheet and leave her on the kitchen table until I got there. In those days, the hazards of aspirin were not known, so the little girl was given one-half of an aspirin tablet.

While driving to the Seidenstecker farm, not only did I get stuck a short distance from their home, I also ran out of a gas. I trudged the short distance from my car to the house on snow shoes, carrying my clinical bag and my burn bag. (I also had a splint bag and a drug bag in those days.)

Ellen woke up as we were assessing the damage. Blistering had already occurred from the back of the knees to the shoulders. Because of the storm and the fact that the family had no hospital insurance, I elected to treat the girl in the home. At that time, Furacin ointment was considered good for burns. I had a supply of that along, as well as sterile dressings, cotton mesh bandages called Kerlix, and elastic bandages sufficient to cover the burn areas with pressure dressings. Several rolls of adhesive tape were applied in spiral fashion to keep the dressings in place. In effect, I created a little mummy.

Oral penicillin from my drug bag was procured from the car along with Empirin No. 3 pills, which were to be cut into quarters and given to the girl every three or four hours, as needed for pain.

Prior to getting some gasoline and helping me get my car

151

out of the snow bank, the Seidenstickers fed me some delicious, freshly-made pork sausage. (They had been in the process of butchering, so the kitchen table had been cleared to make room for Ellen when I told them over the phone what to do.) The meal of fried potatoes and pork sausage were very welcome about 9:30 that night.

For many years thereafter, the homemade summer sausage and occasional pork sausage the Seidensticker family sent us were appreciated by the Albrecht family.

Two weeks later, when we removed the bandages from Ellen, all areas were healed, although the skin was still red. We felt we had really lucked out. It had been a potentially dangerous situation, treated without the benefit of hospitalization.

A little later Laura Seidenstecker was pregnant with her son Ralph and experienced severe toxemia, requiring bed rest and careful attention. Economic factors again played a part in our decision to treat her at home until she was ready to deliver the scrawny infant, who I felt had little chance of survival at birth. We had put Laura and her unborn son in God's hands with prayer during the prenatal care, and I baptized him at birth.

Some weeks later, our two families and the pastor of their church shared a chicken dinner, followed by a confirmation of baptism ceremony. The "scrawny" infant had flourished. We still have a lilac bush given to us that day before we left for home.

One patient of mine actually used my emergency vehicle three times over the five years we provided service. The first time was for a reaction he suffered to one of the herbicides used to treat sweet corn. His wife had taken out his lunch and a thermos of coffee to the field where he was planting corn. The coffee was too hot so without thinking, he used the saucer he had used to put the seed corn into the planter to cool off his coffee. When he became violently ill, I was called.

Emergency care was rendered at home and he was conveyed to the hospital emergency room at West Bend, along with a label from the seed corn bag. We obtained information over the phone from the Poison Control Center in Milwaukee as to how best to proceed and the farmer recovered.

A few years later he survived a coronary which again necessitated a trip in my emergency vehicle. A couple of years after that, a second heart attack made him one patient who needed my emergency vehicle three times. The third time, though, he didn't survive, and left the hospital in the funeral director's vehicle.

It was common in those days to keep a heart attack victim in the hospital for six weeks. We had several oxygen units available to place in the homes of people who might be in need of oxygen, either for a posthospital recuperation, or sometimes for a stroke or heart attack victim we elected to treat without hospitalization.

Between 1952 and 1959, I was the county coroner. Sometimes, it was necessary for Marian to accompany me to the sites of accidents. On occasion, after we loaded the injured into my emergency vehicle, I would perform my coroner duties for the dead and Marian would drive the injured to the hospital. The sheriff or one of his deputies would alert the hospital to have one of my colleagues in West Bend meet her at the emergency room when she arrived. The undertaker who came for the deceased would later drop me off at the hospital. If an autopsy was necessary to determine cause of death, the body was sometimes kept in the hospital morgue until the pathologist arrived. Sometimes the pathologist would go to the funeral home to perform the autopsy.

I recall one two-day period when I was coroner in which, after attempting to resuscitate three drowning victims, I ended up with a back sprain.

For three days I was unable to get off the den floor until my old friend, Dr. Keller, who taught me the principles of osteopathic manipulation, made a home call and got me straightened out.

In 1954 or 1955, the West Bend and Kewaskum Fire Departments requested my help in training their rescue squad personnel. Shortly before I terminated my emergency vehicle service and shortly after I had trained the West Bend firefighters, I had an opportunity to test their newly learned skills and my cardiac massage technique, learned the previous week from Dr. Paul Hausman.

Dr. Hausman had been a local West Bend boy who trained at the Mayo Clinic. He was practicing thoracic surgery in Milwaukee and had come to the West Bend hospital to teach the physicians the principles of both closed and open cardiac resuscitation, using a dog I had anesthetized.

Early one morning, I was called to a home four miles from our place. A little girl of five or six had fallen gravely ill. She had been under the care of a Milwaukee cardiologist for a congenital heart problem. They were waiting for the little girl to grow to a sufficient size to permit cardiac surgery.

When she became ill, the girl's parents called me. Having assessed the problem over the phone, I asked Marian to call the West Bend Fire Department and she gave them directions to the girl's home. By the time they arrived, I was already on the floor of the farm home, trying to oxygenate the unconscious patient with pressure on the bag delivered through an endotracheal tube. There seemed to be some improvement in her color.

When the firefighters arrived, they took over rhythmic pressure on the bag and I started external cardiac massage. After twenty or thirty minutes it was obvious it was a losing battle.

The anguished parents wanted to know if there was anything else we could do. I offered them one last measure of hope. Recalling my session of open cardiac massage training under Dr. Hausman a few weeks earlier, I requested a sharp steak knife.

I opened the girl's chest, and with no other instruments available except my fingers, spread the ribs and massaged the heart. While we didn't resuscitate the little girl, we did achieve a temporary improvement in her color.

Shortly after my emergency vehicle had been acquired, I had a three a.m. call from Charlton Kingsbury, requesting emergency medical care for his wife. Pat was having severe gastrointestinal bleeding both from her mouth and rectum.

I had become acquainted with the Kingsbury family a few months earlier when I was called to their home, about two miles west of Jackson, for their infant daughter Margaret, who had taken ill.

They were in the process of renovating a dilapidated log house that had been vacant for some time. On the earlier visit, I had noted snow sifting through some of the chinks between the logs.

Pat Kingsbury remarked in later years about how impressed she was with my shiny pants, which she described as being almost mirrorlike when I bent over to tend to their child. The suit I wore that day had belonged to the president of the Presbyterian Seminary in Chicago. He had donated it to the American Friends Service Committee for the conscientious objectors at the Merom CPS 14 Camp where I had been some ten years earlier.

In the '50s, people laughed when they recalled the saying popular during the Depression, "God must love the poor because he made so many of us." The night of the hemorrhage, it seemed unlikely Pat would survive to have any further experiences of a hard, but full, life.

When I arrived at the home, it was obvious we had no time to wait. With only itinerant surgeons from Milwaukee available at the Hartford and West Bend hospitals at that time, and limited blood donors for our laboratory nuns to call upon at either hospital, it appeared the best chance for Pat's survival was to take her to Milwaukee Hospital where I had served my

155

internship. While Chuck Kingsbury went to my station wagon to get the stretcher, I called Milwaukee Hospital, requesting they have an emergency surgical staff, laboratory technicians, anesthesiologist and Dr. Donald Thacher ready to go if we arrived with a live patient.

Chuck and I put Pat on the stretcher with a warm blanket from the bed around her and my army blankets around that. We strapped her in, carried her out of the house and placed her in my emergency vehicle. I got the oxygen going.

We said a silent prayer together, hoping she would come back home alive.

I took off with Pat for Milwaukee with red lights flashing and the siren used occasionally to get the few cars ahead of us out of the way. Chuck followed later, after he had made arrangements for someone to care for their children.

Fortunately, everything went like clockwork. Pat lived to experience more trials and tribulations over the ensuing forty years.

Another early morning call to a farm house a few miles south of Jackson resulted in another fast ride to Milwaukee. A visiting relative of the farmer's wife had a ruptured ectopic pregnancy that required the same sort of teamwork and personnel at Lutheran Hospital. (I am not sure when the name changed from Milwaukee to Lutheran Hospital. Many years later, the hospital name was changed again to Sinai-Samaritan).

That emergency call, too, had a successful outcome.

One unsuccessful attempt at trying the impossible happened one afternoon after an auto accident just south of Gumm's Corners. The injured man, in addition to having a skull fracture, was choking to death on his own blood. Unable to get an open airway because of a bilateral fractured jaw, there was no way of getting oxygen to his vital organs. Among my emergency equipment for just such an occasion was a large needle-like cannula, which I introduced into the trachea just below the larynx and hooked up to an oxygen tube which kept him alive until we got to the hospital. It proved to be an exercise in futility. The man died of his injuries.

On a Sunday afternoon early in 1955, a young family from Milwaukee collided with another car which failed to stop for a stop sign on Holy Hill Road where it intersected with the old U.S. Highway 41 (now State Highway 175), south of Jackson. The force of the impact crushed the infant between the mother's body and the dashboard. (Seat belts were not then available in cars.)

The baby was still alive when I arrived at the scene. The mother had a fractured neck and numerous other injuries. As I recall, the father had only a bruised chest. The people responsible for the accident had no injuries.

Among the emergency equipment I carried were wraparound cervical collars. Before we got the lady out of the car, a cervical collar was applied to prevent further damage. Her broken leg was splinted with the help of officers and passersby. We got the baby wrapped up and until we got the mother out of the car, the baby was held by a bystander. The mother was loaded onto the stretcher and placed in my emergency vehicle. The still living baby was placed on her abdomen and covered with blankets. The woman's husband sat on a stool next to the stretcher and we took off with a Washington County Sheriff's Deputy leading the way. Another deputy had been instructed to call ahead to Milwaukee Hospital to have the necessary pediatrician, neurosurgeon and orthopaedic doctors available upon our arrival.

It would be nice to say that all went well, but the baby did not survive. The mother survived, however, and while the family lived in Milwaukee, I had the pleasure of delivering their three children, two boys and a girl, at St. Joseph's Hospital in West Bend. As a memorial to their deceased first born, the family provided St. Joseph's Hospital with pediatric room furniture when their next child was born.

The mother, Anna Fitzer, has had numerous other medical problems and just a few days ago again came out from her Milwaukee home to have a routine exam. There never has been any serious residual effects from the auto accident, but she did correct me to establish the fact that I still had my ambulance in January 1955.

On a Sunday morning in 1954, a farmer living a few miles south of Jackson called me to make an emergency home call on his wife who was having trouble swallowing. When I arrived at the home, I found that the daughter had been under the care of a chiropractor for an obvious polio infection, for which I, as the local health officer for both the village and township of Jackson, should have been informed so I could have placed a quarantine on the house.

It was obvious the mother was suffering from bulbar polio and that she soon would need an iron lung. To be eligible for an iron lung or, indeed for a hospital room, in those years of scarcity, it was necessary to prove patients had polio before they were admitted. Such proof required, in addition to clinical findings and history, a spinal tap for analysis. The practice then at St. Joseph's Hospital in West Bend was to use a room adjacent to the ambulance entrance and across from the morgue for purposes of doing the spinal tap and watching the patient while the laboratory confirmed the diagnosis before admitting the patient. Our three iron lungs were all in service and none of the Milwaukee hospitals had an iron lung available. The University Hospitals in Madison had one unoccupied iron lung, which I could have for my patient as soon as the lab confirmed the diagnosis.

During the time of waiting to confirm the obvious, I went up to my anesthesia machine and took off the 100 cc. aspirating syringe as well as some of my other anesthetic equipment so that on our trip to Madison I might be able to remove fluid from my patient's airway.

Both the patient and her husband were apprehensive, as I was. I agreed wholeheartedly with their request that we make arrangements for her to have communion before going to Madison. Fortunately, their pastor was able to meet us at the corner of State Highways 45 and 60 on the way to Madison. In the front yard of a church of another denomination, we met and prayed together. My patient was unable to swallow but did taste the elements before we started for Madison.

Before leaving their house, I had aspirated mucus from her mouth and pharynx. Before we got to Hartford, it was obvious that even though we had asked God with believing hearts that she survive, the issue was very much in doubt. I pulled into the yard of St. Joseph's Hospital in Hartford (now called Hartford Memorial), where I was still a member of the active staff and giving anesthesia. Before going into the hospital, I aspirated the patient once more. I left her in the care of her husband and asked Sister Joseph at the admitting desk to please call the sheriff to provide me with an escort to Madison. I then suctioned the patient again, reassured her that I thought we would get there in time, and took off.

We picked up our deputy escort about a mile west of Hartford. Despite my siren and red lights, Sunday drivers persisted in getting out of the way for the squad car but would get back on the road in front of my vehicle. Traveling at seventy and seventy-five miles an hour made this a precarious ride. A curve a couple miles west of Hartford almost proved our undoing when we hit the shoulder and swerved erratically. After that, we cut the speed to a more reasonable sixty-five. The Washington County Sheriff's Department communicated with Dodge County and Columbia County, so that we were escorted at a more reasonable speed the rest of the way to Madison.

As we approached Columbus, more than half way to Madison, a gurgling sound resembling a death rattle impelled me to pull off the road to do a little more professional job of aspirating the woman than her husband had been able to accomplish. He was still white, recalling the near catastrophe forty-five minutes earlier. I suspect I probably wasn't much better.

It seemed as though we probably wouldn't make it to Madison unless we changed places so that I could keep her airway open. I asked him if he could drive. He stated he could drive but he didn't know where to drive to. I told him I would give him directions as we went along. So we changed places, got through Columbus, then through Sun Prairie, and onto Johnson Street and University Avenue in Madison, the back way to the university's Orthopaedic Hospital where the iron lung was located.

The patient recovered and came home ten days later. She survives to this day and is still my patient.

My colleague, Dr. Ralph Olsen, a year or so ago reminded me how we met. In 1954 he was a resident in pediatrics at the University of Wisconsin Hospitals during one of the last polio epidemics before the advent of Salk vaccine. He mentioned how impressed he was that a country doctor would bring a patient to the hospital in his own emergency vehicle.

21

"Coroner, 1952 to 1959 "

I n the 1940s and '50s, even though physicians were busy, it was felt we had a professional obligation to provide community service outside the realm of treating the ill.

As a community responsibility, I felt I should be involved, not only working with the county nurse in the immunization programs and acting as the local health officer, but also assuming the position of county coroner, even though the statutes did not require the coroner had to be a physician. My friend, Dr. Frankow, had earlier been coroner and had been replaced by Dr. Richard Driessel, who in 1952 decided he had had enough. The chairman of the county's Republican Party prevailed on me to run for the elected post. Since Washington County historically has been a Republican stronghold, I couldn't lose the election, even if the Democrats could find a candidate! I didn't.

I still can't understand how I could spread myself so thin, to the detriment of my family.

My time as coroner coincided with my realization of the deleterious affects alcohol had on the lives of my patients and society. Auto accidents to which I was called as coroner, many times were obviously related to drinking. Neither the coroner's nor the sheriff's report forms had a place to record that fact until the mid-1950s, when the Coroners Association rectified the omission. It was only natural that as I investigated these fatalities, that I would become active in changing the status quo.

Imagine the shock of finding three young men dead in the front seat of a car. They had been traveling west on County Highway K, just east of the then new U.S. Highway 41, when a drunken youth collided with them head-on. All three young men had broken necks and bruised foreheads from hitting the windshield on impact.

That experience impelled me to have a safety belt installed in the front seat of my emergency vehicle and in my personal cars years before seatbelts became a standard feature.

Another experience, where a young man burning to death in the back seat of a car which left the road and rolled over several times before it caught fire, was a sight — and smell — I will never forget.

Empty beer bottles, whiskey and brandy bottles littered the shoulders of the highways and were commonly found under the seats of cars involved in fatal accidents. Members of society felt that what they did with their lives was of no concern to anyone except themselves and that they knew when to draw the line. The beer and alcohol interests had powerful lobbyists in Madison. The voices for temperance and controlled drinking, by comparison, were few and weak. Many couldn't understand that if they were old enough at eighteen to fight and die for their country, why shouldn't they be allowed to drink alcoholic beverages? Underage drinking accounted for a disproportionate share of the highway accidents and fatalities. The Coroners Association was instrumental in having both the coroner's report and the sheriff's report have specific places to enter observed evidence of the involvement of alcohol in accidents.

Statewide attention was drawn to a neighboring county when a car, full of drunken youths coming home from a teenage bar, was involved in a grisly accident. One of the inebriated young men stuck his head out the window on the passenger side of the car. The car swerved too close to a fixed mailbox on the roadside resulting in decapitation.

Alcohol was then beginning to be recognized as a disease. My involvement in fighting that disease will be discussed in another chapter. These few incidents involving alcohol related deaths in this recall of my days as coroner are sufficient. There is little purpose in pursuing this point when there are so many other recollections of my experiences as coroner.

I apologize for this seemingly schizophrenic approach to the narrative. It is hard to plainly separate the tapestry of one's life experiences into neat compartments. The subject of this chapter covers the entire panorama of the end of life necessitating the coroner's attention.

In the past forty years, the pace of life and death has quickened. People of today have become so accustomed to details of violence and death that I fear that this account of a more leisurely paced generation will be boring.

The time I am recalling in this chapter, 1952 to 1959, had its share of tragedies much less widely sensationalized than is common today.

The gruesome details of suicide and murder, as well as the details of the deaths in industry and home, have become so commonplace that we tend to think in generic terms and react in generic ways, in a "So What!" fashion. We don't think of identifying ourselves with either the deceased or the survivors.

I can't recall a time when I was called to either an accident scene as a physician-ambulance driver or when called to the scene as a coroner that I failed to ask God to help me do what He would have me do and not "make an ass of myself." Once at the scene, my efforts were to do what should be done. When a life was gone, those at the scene, either survivors, bystanders or helpers, were invited to participate in a moment of prayer for the soul of the deceased, and for the peace and comfort of his or her survivors.

Never was I able to answer the question, "Why did God permit this to happen?" When addressing the questions inevitable at the time of serious injury or death, contributing causes can be postulated, but the innermost thoughts of the deceased, as well as of the survivors, are known but to God.

The individual experiences of each of us in life, as in death, is nicely summarized in the brief statement attributed to Kahil Gibran: "Whereas each of us is alone in the knowledge of God, so is each of us alone in his knowledge of God and His understanding of the earth." I was never able to satisfactorily understand why the incident to be related now ever occurred.

Five or six weeks prior to the birth of our son Charles, a coroner's call to a car-train wreck a few miles south of Jackson involved one of the three or four such fatal collisions during my tenure as coroner. The deceased apparently didn't see the train coming from the south, or tried to cross ahead of it, and was hit. The car was demolished and thrown three or four hundred feet to the north of the point of impact. The body was pretty badly mangled, but with the help of the undertaker, we got together most of the pieces.

Unfortunately, I wasn't as attentive to where I was walking as I should have been and inadvertently straddled the tow rope running from the tow truck's winch to the major portion of the demolished car. As the line became taut, the angle was such that it forcibly impacted on my crotch, causing considerable immediate agony and within ten or twelve hours, sufficient hematoma and severe pain to necessitate seven or eight days of hospitalization for treatment of bilateral orchitis.

I was indebted to Dr. William C. P. Hoffman of Hartford to help hold my practice together by coming to my office during my hospitalization. Within a two week period we had succeeded in getting a locum tenens, Dr. Harry Evans, to join me temporarily while I recuperated over the next six weeks.

Due to the accident, Chuck was the only one of our three children at whose birth I was able to be present. I have since learned there are less traumatic forms of birth control!

Murder-suicide was not as common then, as now. I recall only one case that sticks vividly in my mind. This event occurred near the southernmost border of Washington County. The Sheriff's Department had been notified by relatives that they had not been able to contact the deceased by telephone. The deceased's German shepherds were hungry when the relatives went to the house to investigate. Apparently there had been some marital problems that the relatives were aware of, and I expect they suspected what the Sheriff's Department found and reported to me as coroner. When I arrived, it was obvious that a mere doctor would be of no help.

We never did determine the "why," but it was apparent from the physical evidence that the "how" was a gunshot wound in the head of each, with the woman shot in the head as she knelt to the right of the bed. Her companion knelt to her right and also was shot in the head, the gun under his lifeless hand.

In later years, while no longer coroner, one of my patients involved in a marital triangle died by the hand of the aggrieved husband who shot both his wife and her lover in their home. Some weeks later, the husband was found, a suicide by drowning, in Lake Michigan.

My hat goes out to the grandmother of their two children, as well as to the children themselves. The grandmother is a great person, a widow whose husband had died some years earlier of a cerebral aneurysm. (By this time I think my readers are aware that I have had personal relationships with my patients and that each was a friend as well as a professional obligation.) This is probably a reaction to my own experience at the time of my father's death.

One-car accidents, usually caused by inattentive driving, alcohol-related stupidity or an unfamiliar road conditions such as icy bridges accounted for a disproportionate share of all auto accidents. Mechanical error or defect was a factor in some. The relatively late development of seat belts as a standard feature in most road vehicles substantially decreased the incidents of certain types of injury but inattentive attitude on the part of many motorists who think, "It can't happen to me," is still instrumental in causing many unnecessary deaths and injuries to both driver and passenger.

During the seven years I was coroner there were perhaps ten or twelve deaths of either drivers or passengers thrown from their vehicles as the doors buckled on the force of impact against other vehicles or immovable objects, or even by the blowout of a tire causing loss of control.

Carbon monoxide deaths were particularly hard to ascribe to either accident or suicide. Most often, it was apparent that termination of life was the primary goal. If the deaths occurred, as they often did, with the car running in an isolated area until it ran out of gas, and we found a hose connected to the exhaust pipe with the other end running into a partially open window, there was no question. If it happened in a closed garage and the persons alcohol content was above 0.15 or 0.20, there might be a reasonable doubt. I am not sure how life insurance companies made the determination when it involved double indemnity.

Death by ingestion of toxic substances was a little more difficult to explain prior to the advent of forensic pathologists. Unless there was obvious clear-cut evidence, some of these may have been missed in establishing the actual cause of death. One exception was the occasional corpse with the characteristic cyanide odor (odor of oil of bitter almonds).

A person whose lips and mouth were burned and who died an agonizing death in a very short time, and who had an open lye can next to the body left no questions as to the "how." The questions "why," and "when" many times were left unanswered. The agony on the face of the deceased gave me the impression that this was not the way to go.

Self-inflicted gunshot wounds were probably more common in Washington County in the 1950s than death by gunshot inflicted by others, either accidently or intentionally. Head wounds probably were more common, more messy and probably caused more anguish to the family than gunshot wounds to the heart, the manner chosen by my father to end his life.

Self-inflicted stab wounds causing death were less common. If the method chosen was to cut a major artery, many times help arrived in time to stop the bleeding. Then the ethical question arose as to whether one gave transfusions to preserve the life that the person so desperately wanted to end. Occasionally the brush with death reversed the desire to die, but I recall several instances where subsequent attempts by more lethal means fulfilled the death wish.

Death by hanging in a barn or garage were not uncommon. There were occasional deaths by hanging in bathrooms, where the body blocked the door, necessitating someone to crawl through a window and cut the body down to enable the door to be opened. Regardless of where the event took place, this form of death probably was the most painful since seldom was the neck broken, and the death came as a result of strangulation.

Death by over-use of alcohol to achieve a blood level much above the legal limit of intoxication were not uncommon in those years. Deaths were either purposeful or unintentional. Self-overdosage of prescription drugs were less common. Occasionally, one could question, but never prove, whether the refusal of an individual to take medication as prescribed leading to death was willful or accidental. At least on the death certificate and in my heart, I gave the deceased the benefit of the doubt.

My resignation as coroner was necessitated by the realization that service to the living with alcohol problems was more important than service to the dead. I also needed to continue treating the people I had come to Jackson to serve. With my resignation ended the tradition of a physician as coroner in Washington County.

22

"Visions
and
Dreams"

"Your old men shall dream dreams, your young men shall see visions." Job 2:28.

At the age of seventy-seven, I qualify to have the dreams of an old man. I have never been accused of acting my age, so possibly I can qualify as being a young visionary also!

January 1, 1993, was the forty-ninth anniversary of my first date with Marian. On December 10, 1992, friends and visitors paid their respects to Marian at the Schmidt Funeral Home in Jackson. Friends from far and near admired twenty-five or thirty of her paintings, expertly put on exhibit at the funeral home by our friends from the West Bend Gallery of Fine Arts. Many of our friends were amazed at the versatile nature of her paintings and suggested that reprints be made available before I dispose of the originals.

A few years ago, Marian had painted for our daughter Lynn Vegafria a beautiful sunset view of the outdoor worship center overlooking Mission Lake Church Camp, where we spent many happy family vacations over the years. Lynn had lent the picture to me for this postmortem show.

Mission Lake camping friends, who had come from far and near to pay their respects, also had fond remembrances of that particular lake scene. They liked the painting, which had been publicly displayed only for one month two years earlier at the 1990 Washington County Artists annual exhibition.

One of Marian's last watercolors, completed only three or four days before her stroke, was a picture of the home of our friends Lawrence and Monica Plaskan. They had not yet picked it up at the time of her death. The Plaskan's graciously allowed me to display this painting above Marian's very first watercolor, created for our granddaughter Cora. Rather than using her usual signature, "Marian Albrecht" with the year it was painted, for Cora's painting, she signed it "Grandma."

When I delivered Marian's last painting to the Plaskan's on New Year's Eve day, they reminded me that they had one of her 1989 masterpieces, which I fondly remembered when they showed it to me. The Plaskans graciously offered to allow me to use Marian's original painting of the old Washington County Courthouse and Jail, now the home of the Washington County Historical Society and historical buildings in their own right, for reprints.

Eleven years ago, Marian and I formed a business partnership we called Painter & Potter. Over the last several years, Marian and I were invited to participate in the Washington County Historical Society's annual art show held on the museum grounds. At these shows, I would often remember visits with the sheriff and the people who had worked at the old jailhouse while I was county coroner many years earlier.

These two paintings, the county buildings and Mission Lake sunset, and five other paintings representative of Marian's work, are the nucleus for a series of prints I am producing, with profits earmarked for the benefit of church camps and the Washington County Historical Society. The proceeds of my autobiography have been dedicated to help provide ongoing support for the work of Lutheran Social Services long after we both have left this life.

The support of family, friends, colleagues and patients after Marian's death has been deeply appreciated. It has also been consoling to me to recognize that Marian's relatively rapid and painless death was a blessing compared to the long, lingering death she might have had.

Twelve or fourteen years ago, while Marian was still working in my office, my long-time assistant, Dolores Mayer, suggested to her how much less traumatic it would be for the survivor if we had our headstone installed prior to one of us dying. Some years earlier, we had purchased a lot at our church cemetery. Both of us realized that it was only a matter of time before that lot would be used. We visited several cemeteries, but found no stones that appealed to both of us.

As we were eating at Heidel's Restaurant outside Jackson one noon, the restaurant's owner, Wayne Heidel, a friend of our's, suggested we might wish to consult with his son-in-law, Walter Miller, who worked for the West Bend Monument Company, a branch of Hilgendorf Memorial of Cedarburg. When none of the catalogues showed exactly what we had in mind, Wally suggested Marian draw a diagram of the form we wished. A few days later, he returned to our dining room with a cardboard replica of her sketch. The form was right, but the size was much too large. It was cut down to a less ostentatious size.

We visited the plant a couple of times while the stone was

being cut. Over the years since the gravestone was installed, we would visit the cemetery. Knowledge of the inevitability of death and the remembrance of these things made the Christmas after Marian's death less traumatic for me.

A shared vision some years ago was fulfilled that Christmas. A Christmas wreath sufficiently large to encircle the names on the monument and with cut boughs covering the frozen ground was placed over her grave.

The third thing which made this time of bereavement bearable is the fact that Marian planned her own funeral long before her final illness. The only deviation from her written plan was the beautiful music provided by our long-time friends Alice Stauss on the harpsichord and Ann Marie Rath-Schowalter on the cello, in a prelude to the worship at her funeral.

Not wishing to have our relatives miss the musical prelude to the worship, I insisted on another deviation: That relatives be permitted to remain seated during the final moments before the casket was closed instead of being ushered out, as is usually the case, before joining the procession prior to the funeral service. I am glad we did and commend that arrangement to others.

I think the only thing we had not yet accomplished prior to her death, but had spoken of for a couple years, was the relatively new concept of a prearranged funeral in which we would have both selected a coffin and other funeral arrangements while we were still living. Both of us had the difficult experience of arranging funerals at the times of death of grandparents, parents, uncles and aunts. Yet we did not take the time to organize our own funeral plans ahead of time. I appreciated our children and grandchildren helping in the arrangements for Marian.

Each family must make their own decision from the standpoint of economics, but it makes sense to make the investment some years before inflation will have substantially increased the cost. As I understand it, preplanned funeral funds are invested in a trust, with the interest on the investment supposedly sufficient to offset inflationary changes.

It is my hope that by sharing these experiences and reflections, at least some of my readers will be able to more realistically accept the inevitable loss of a loved one with greater equanimity than had I not shared my experience.

CHAPTER

23

"AA and Al-Anon in Washington County"

O ne rainy April morning, about 5:30, five-year-old Lynn came into our bedroom somewhat worried with a complaint. "There is a man smoking in our bathroom," she said.

We reassured her we knew about the man and that there was nothing to be concerned about.

Frank had come to our door about 11:30 the previous evening requesting help. I had met him earlier and was aware that his family had thrown him out because of chronic alcoholism. Being mindful of the admonition, "Whatsoever you have done to the least of these, My brethren, you have done also unto Me," Marian and I gave him something to eat, a blanket and a cot. I am not certain what happened to him after we gave him breakfast, but I think Frank went to the Rescue

Mission in Milwaukee. He eventually died a few years later.

Following that experience, we left unlocked the outer door of the waiting room. This had been converted from an old porch on the north side of the house into a gas-heated waiting room with a locked door leading into the business office. Somewhat surprisingly, none of the homeless who utilized that area during cold weather abused the privilege. Friends and relatives were somewhat upset at our reliance on the goodness of human nature.

A few years later, after we had built our present home and moved in the fall of 1956, we had another similar occurrence. A man who had been raised in the Jackson area drove off the road into a swamp about eight miles away. He walked to our home, requesting help. He became one of my success stories during the era I was coroner.

Assisting my great uncle Art Butterbrodt and my brother Harry in committing my uncle Walde, who was also my godfather, to the Winnebago State Mental Hospital in 1953 affected me greatly. I developed a vendetta against the effects of alcohol on the lives of people. Within a week of that harrowing experience with my uncle, while attending services at my wife's home church where we had been married nine years earlier, I was favorably impressed by the sermon presented by Rev. Ernst Parrish, head of the United Temperance Movement of Wisconsin. He likened alcoholism to an infectious disease, with the germ of that disease being alcohol itself. At that time, it was thought that one of every fifteen people who drank socially would develop a problem with alcohol, sooner or later. In recent years, that statistic gradually has increased to a ratio of about one in ten.

Rev. Parrish asked how many of us in the congregation would feel free to imbibe from a bottle with a pretty label containing a substance which might temporarily make us feel good, knowing that we contributed to the well-being of the country and state by paying a tax on the contents. However, he said, if there was a one in fifteen chance of contracting diphtheria, whooping cough, scarlet fever, tuberculosis or a venereal disease, would we still be willing to take that chance?

Those were words I could understand. I surprised myself by writing a check for one hundred dollars to the United Temperance Movement on the spot. As a consequence, I was invited to become a member of the organization and eventually became an officer for a number of years. I went to Madison to testify before legislative committees about the effects of alcohol on society in general, as well as on the people who came to my attention as coroner.

After one of those appearances, the local sheriff had a telephone call one morning from a television station asking what he thought about the testimony in Madison the day before by the Washington County coroner. The sheriff was quoted on TV that night, saying, "What does Dr. Albrecht know about alcoholism? He is only an alcoholic himself."

One of my physician friends from Milwaukee called to let me know this was a clear case of libel, and that he was sending a hundred dollar donation for me to use as the start of a legal fund to sue the sheriff for everything he had. When I called the sheriff, who I had always considered a friend, he sputtered some and indicated that he had been caught off guard while he was shaving, and that he was sorry.

I asked him to put that apology in writing and not to let it happen again. While I probably did have cause for action against him, I wouldn't have felt right about pursuing the matter further.

During the 1950s, I felt like a lone voice crying in the wilderness. Some of my patients had medical problems of which alcohol was either a primary or contributing cause. I soon developed a reputation for having a soft spot in my heart for families with alcohol problems in one or the other spouses, usually the male.

I developed a habit of seeing the husband and wife together at the time of the first appointment so that there was no question in either's mind as to what the doctor said or did. I adopted the principles of developing a mutual trust and reliance on God to direct our efforts at helping the family. Being a realist, I would tell the family, "I am not going to charge you in dollars because you can't possibly pay me what it will be worth for you to stop drinking. However, after you have been dry for six months, I will expect you to answer the call I may direct to you at any time of the night or day to help someone else who has a problem with alcohol."

By the time I resigned as coroner in 1959, I had perhaps fifteen or twenty families practicing sobriety with this somewhat unorthodox approach.

A pastor from Cedarburg called me early one Monday morning, indicating he had an unemployed parishioner who had been in DTs — delirium tremens, the painful, physical symptoms of alcohol withdrawal, including convulsive seizures (the "shakes") — since the previous night and didn't look good. The pastor brought the parishioner, whose name was Stanley, and Stanley's wife to my office.

It was obvious Stanley was very likely to die if he didn't get immediate attention. We started an intravenous line in the office as we evaluated the situation. We gave Stanley some medication along with the intravenous solution.

The Sister Superior at St. Joseph's Hospital was called. She was told I didn't think the hospital would ever get paid, but that Stanley would die if we didn't give him care. I thought the nursing care could be limited because I could have friends come in to sit with him until Stanley was over his shakes.

She agreed to take him.

I got on the phone and talked to two of the families who "owed me." I explained that I needed four people to stay with Stanley night and day until he was over the DTs. I assigned each of them to call two other people and make arrangements for that coverage.

It took Stanley four days to recover enough where he didn't have to have constant surveillance. Within two weeks, his blood chemistry returned close enough to normal so that we could send him home. In another two weeks Stanley's boss gave him his job back on the basis of my telephone call.

It would be nice to be able to say that Stanley was one of my successes, but about two years later Stanley relapsed and died of complications from the liver damage caused by his alcohol abuse. He was one of the relatively few I had contact with who didn't maintain sobriety.

By this time, the judges in the county had learned about my interest in alcoholism and frequently asked me to see people before the judges had to make the decision to send them to Winnebago State Hospital — where the treatment had not greatly improved since we put uncle Walde there seven years earlier. In addition, employers were beginning to realize that recovering alcoholics deserved a chance at rehabilitation. Many times, I would call and say that mister so-and-so was under my care, had been dry for six months, and that I felt he had an eighty-five percent chance of remaining dry, would you please give him another chance? Often they did.

But for all its success, it became apparent that our recovery program needed something more than my prescribed initial prayer of supplication, repeated prayers of thanksgiving during the period of observation, and the Librium or Valium to be taken instead of alcohol when the urge became too great. We had heard of Alcoholics Anonymous. There was a branch of AA at Hartford, as well as in Milwaukee, where Allis Chalmers had become an enlightened employer, recognizing the need for a social outlet as well as ongoing concern for the recovering alcoholic and his family.

The local social custom of the time for many people involved spending Saturday nights at a tavern, many times both husband and wife going together. The thought occurred to me that I could kill two birds with one stone by offering a social gathering at my office Saturday nights, and thus was born AA and Al-Anon in Jackson.

My patients and friends invited a few members of the small AA group in Hartford, as well as Reverend Ralph Maschmeier, pastor of Peace United Church of Christ. Pastor Maschmeier was the first of many pastors to encourage our efforts, and one of the few to attend our early meetings.

Peace United Church had been located at the corner of State Highways 45 and 60 in Jackson. A branch office of the West Bend Savings Bank and Dairy Queen have replaced the parsonage and church.

The local population soon spoke derisively of "Doc's Club." But many times, we had thirty-nine people attend on Saturday nights, overloading my little office. Village officials then allowed us to use the basement of the Village Hall, where twelve years earlier I had agreed to come to Jackson.

After a few months there, it became apparent that this was not a warm enough environment to keep the people coming.

In late winter or early spring, Christ Lutheran Church, of which I was a member, had a special meeting to address some other church issue. When that was resolved, I asked permission to speak to the group about a problem close to my heart. I asked if they would offer the church's Fellowship Hall on Saturday evenings for the meetings of my alcoholic friends.

There was a protest that I was out of order. It became apparent that few, if any, were very enthusiastic about my proposal. The impression was, "Those drunken bums will damage our church."

I pointed out that I was prepared to compensate the church for any damage my friends may do, but I still hadn't made a sale. In that era, the contribution of each church member was publicized at the time of the annual meeting. Marian and I had tithed from the time of our marriage and went somewhat over the usual ten percent so that the published amount of our contribution for the past year was substantially greater than a third of the total church budget for the previous year.

When I got up again, my final statement was to the effect that if my friends could not use the Fellowship Hall on Saturday nights, even if I compensated for any damage they might do, I really couldn't see how my wife and I could continue to worship with such "saintly" people on Sunday mornings.

The message was well received and my proposal unanimously carried. Needless to say, my AA groups and Al-Anon did a better job of taking care of the church than many of the church groups that also met there. Sometimes, our Saturday evening congregation in Fellowship Hall exceeded in numbers the Sunday morning worship numbers!

We had our ups and down. At one point the question arose as to why Dr. Albrecht, who was not an alcoholic, could attend meetings and have so much to say about the group. In response, some of the members pointed out that without Dr. Albrecht there would be no place to meet and that, at times, the meetings would not have very many participants at all if Dr. Albrecht wasn't there, too. I think I have the distinction of being the only person elected "honorary alcoholic" in the state.

Our little group in Jackson grew and developed daughter groups as far away as Green Bay, ninety miles north, as well as in Ozaukee County and in West Bend.

By 1968, citizens such as Father Jerome Ziegler, Dr. F. I. Bush, Dr. James Baumgartner, Bill Rock, as well as some of the lawyers, members of the clergy, law enforcement officials and Social Service people, came to realize that a more formal organization was necessary to address the problems of alcoholism in the county. Informal discussions resulted in a feasibility study for the proposal of forming an Alcohol Problems Council, which I believe was finalized sometime in 1970.

By that time, I was embarked on the next challenge God arranged for me through extraordinary circumstances, the development of the Drug Information Center of Washington County in 1970.

24

"Washington County Drug Council"

Not long ago, Sue Calhoun, a long-time friend and former employee who still comes to my home to keep my records properly straightened and filed, was here to get things in order for the next visit of my current professional management counselor, John Miller. She found records I didn't know existed any more, papers that have helped me focus more clearly on some of the events of my life for this book than would have been possible by memory alone. One of those records is a letter I wrote on March 27, 1972.

In the interest of presenting an orderly progression of my involvement in the treatment of substance abuse locally, I submit a version of that letter I wrote to then President Richard M. Nixon.

President Richard M. Nixon
The White House
Washington, D.C.

Dear President Nixon:

This letter is being sent at the suggestion of my professional management counselor, Mr. Paul R. Miller of Madison, Wisconsin, when we were discussing over lunch your attempts to marshall the resources of our country to combat the drug menace. We are grateful for your efforts. Mr. Miller thought you would be interested in some of the experiences we've had in Washington County relating to drugs and alcohol.

For twelve years I have been working with alcoholics in our community as a part of my general practice. At the onset, I encouraged some of my patients to start an AA group which first met in my office, and then in a local church. Subsequently, these alcoholics and their spouses have been instrumental in starting several other AA and Al-Anon groups.

Initially, in return for my professional help and personal involvement, each new patient was requested to agree that part of my recompense would be the ability, after he had achieved sobriety for six months, to be on call to help others with a similar problem. This principle of "Christianity in action" has remained the cornerstone of our official program, and the arrested alcoholic has found help for himself as he helps others to achieve and maintain sobriety.

Unfortunately we do not have statistics, but [we] have worked with over 750 alcoholics with a good degree of success. We have had the cooperation and endorsement of the local medical society from the time we started, and have had good communication with the Department of Social Services, the Guidance Center, members of the clergy, the county judges, law enforcement officials, and the attorneys. Employers have been helpful, and many men who have lost their jobs have regained them.

There has been a great satisfaction in seeing the self-respect of people who have been on welfare for years finally achieving economic stability for themselves and families through [the] maintenance of sobriety.

This work has been done without cost to the state or federal government, and the only cost to local governments is the occasional person who has been incarcerated or committed as an alcoholic before accepting treatment, or those who have had relapse.

Our local daily paper, the *West Bend News*, has run a free advertisement in the personal column ever since we have started, giving my telephone number and the telephone numbers of members of AA to call if persons have immediate problems. We call appropriate AA members for immediate referral, refer the complicated case to the appropriate social agency or hospital, and for those who need medical attention, either take care of them in our office or at the local hospital, or refer them to their own physician.

Over the years there has developed a community recognition of the fact that we do have a problem with alcohol, and in July of this year a group of interested citizens met in West Bend to discuss formation of a Washington County Council on Alcoholism.

The previous week, the young college-bound son of one of my laboratory technician friends, had ventilated to his mother about the lack of social concern of members of the establishment as regards to drugs and the youth culture. He said to his mother, who conveyed the message to me, "If Dr. Albrecht can do so much for the alcoholic, why can't he or someone else take an interest in and do something for the kids with drug problems?"

When this question was brought to me by his mother, I remembered instances of drug abuse in our community, and was aware that various people in the establishment were saying something should be done, but no one knew exactly what to do or what the extent of the problem was. There was nothing except concern and limited action on the part of the law enforcement officials. Episodic care of individuals by the physicians or the Guidance Center led to the recognition of the increasing problem. Defense attorneys, prosecuting attorneys, district attorney, judges and society in general were concerned but didn't know what could be done.

Discussions are good, but action must follow. This young man's suggestion and challenge was brought to the attention of the [people at the Washington County Council on Alcoholism] meeting, with the suggestion made that we bring into the proposed new council, with its dreams for a hot line and information center, the problem of drugs. Initially this was thought well of, but subsequently, the people who have had experience with alcoholics felt they would have no rapport with the drug problem.

Five or six of the people at that meeting went to Madison the following week for a training session on contributions needed to address the problem of substance abuse. Many are presently enrolled in a course on alcoholic counseling at the local high school, and the group is contemplating incorporation.

The following Sunday morning, I had a twelve-year-old boy and a fourteen-year-old girl admitted as an emergency to our local hospital with drug intoxication. I felt impelled, as the collection plate was passed in Christ Lutheran Church, to write a note to the pastor asking for a few minutes of time with the congregation following the service. This was granted, and I made the plea to the congregation for help in developing community support.

Several people responded, both adults and young people. Word got around that the Council on Alcoholism decided not to have anything to do with drugs. Several mothers and interested young people approached me. They have done all of the work and study, and have incorporated as the Washington County Council on Drug Information. Thirty-one [volunteers] have started or are well on the way toward completion of an eight-week course designed to make them able to answer hot line [calls], and to talk with people who call. Referral sources are being contacted, and as soon as the IRS approval is given to the organization, funds will be solicited.

In the meantime, one of our local banks has lent the group $1,250 to finance the course for those interested. A small room in the West Bend Library will be utilized initially until finances and more commodious quarters make expansion possible.

It is good to see the spirit of cooperation between the generations in seeking a solution and jointly working together in achieving a solution of the problem, which affects all of society. Ultimately we may appeal for assistance from the government, but it is our philosophy that it is better to try to get started with local support, make use of as much volunteer help as we can, so that the people involved will have the satisfaction of helping one another toward a common goal. We are hopeful that by establishing communication between the generations [and] by offering understanding and help, we may prevent many young people from trying drugs, and be able to help those who have tried them to avoid disastrous complications and consequences.

It seems to me that no matter how much money is invested in a program, to be successful it must have broad community support and interested citizen participation. While we can't claim to have achieved success, we do feel there is promise in the work of the interested citizens of Washington County, and hope these experiences might be utilized to make more effective the work under your direction.

Sincerely yours,
James Albrecht, MD

cc to: Glenn R. Davis, Congressman
       Wm. A. Steiger, Congressman
       Gaylord Nelson, U.S. Senator
       Wm. Proxmire, U.S. Senator

PS: Is there any possibility of proclaiming the National Day of Prayer for 1972 several weeks ahead of the appointed date, and requesting the news media and the people of this country to join in a concerted effort of prayer to Almighty God to lead and guide all of us as instruments of His peace; that He may continue to guide our nation, its leaders and people in the paths which He would have us follow? Thank you for the consideration of this letter.

Paul R. Miller, mentioned in the first paragraph, had been my professional management counselor since 1953. When he became ill, he arranged for his son John to continue in his stead. When Paul died, the family requested I deliver the eulogy. As I have said, friendly, personal relationships are all important in having a happy life. The reference in the postscript to the possibility of proclaiming a National Day of Prayer for 1972 several weeks ahead of the appointed date will be explained in chapter26.

Despite the copies to our Senators and Representatives, I am unaware, unlike my earlier letter regarding the National Day of Prayer, that this letter had any effect on the drug problem, which has continued to escalate far beyond what we visualized twenty-one years ago.

I am happy to report, though, that for some years now, my initial dream of combining the drug and alcohol programs locally has been consummated, with the formation of the Council on Alcohol and Other Drug Abuse of Washington County.

Yet, it is disappointing that our efforts have not been more successful in slowing the deterioration of society. We did try our best.

25

"Detours Along the Way"

Besides practicing medicine full time and continuing the practice of anesthesia part time until the mid-'70s, I became involved with peripheral interests that I will mention briefly.

One day at Hartford Hospital, I was giving anesthesia to a critically ill woman undergoing surgery for a ruptured ectopic pregnancy. A relatively light, stainless steel intravenous stand was being used for the procedure. We had extended the stand's support arm to its maximum height, to increase the flow of blood and intravenous fluids and maintain adequate blood pressure in the patient.

Somehow, the stand tipped over, to the consternation of not only the anesthesiologist, but of the surgeons and nurses. While the patient survived, the rest of us in the operating room had some bad moments until the situation was rectified.

That incident inspired me. Over the next year and a half, I developed a prototype anesthesia table with an attached intravenous stand capable of safely extending its support arm to seven and one half feet. The arm could rotate a full three hundred and sixty degrees and had four hooks, giving the attending anesthetist or anesthesiologist a wide latitude of treatment options, as well as the ability to hang intravenous fluids in advance of the next case. My design helped minimize wasted time between cases, keeping the operating room team on schedule.

After I found that my prototype intravenous stand worked, a side venture, called the Ora Table Company — with an ox yolk for its registered trade mark — took up my spare time, both in development and distribution. It was never a very successful business, although we did eventually sell tables in forty-eight states. Ultimately, the cost of production escalated from two hundred and forty dollars for each stand to seven hundred and eighty dollars in 1978, the year before the Shah of Iran was deposed.

By that time, I also had developed a padded aluminum arm board with Velcro straps to maintain an anesthetized patient's arm in a position of comfort while being stabilized to prevent inadvertent motion from dislodging an intravenous needle. While this was a good idea and practical at the time, the development of the intravenous catheter at about the same time made the Ora arm board obsolete before it got off the ground.

This side venture almost ended in disaster. It was the impetus to finance an ill-fated tool and die company, Rectangle Tool and Die, which expired in a couple of years, teaching me an expensive lesson.

This lesson was probably directed by God to force me to remain active instead of retiring at the age of sixty-five as I had originally visualized. In retrospect, I would have been miserable retired, and probably would have jumped from the frying pan into the fire in some other fashion.

In 1973 I was made a fellow of the American Academy of Family Practice, of which I was a charter member. The ceremony was held in Denver, Colorado, and we took a side trip to the mountains north of Blackhawk and Central City, where we bought an acre lot for a retirement home. This project became a near catastrophe, and we wasted a lot of time and effort over the next several years as we tried to build our own Shangri-la.

Wisconsin to Colorado was too great a distance to adequately supervise the project. What started out as a thirty-two thousand dollar vacation house, turned into a seventy-six thousand dollar, two-story home. To add insult to financial injury, just before the completion of the home, the year of the great Thompson River flood, it was vandalized to the extent of more than twenty thousand dollars. Fortunately, the loss was covered by construction insurance, because the dishwasher, stove and refrigerator had not yet been installed, but had been vandalized in the crates.

The home had windows on three sides of the upper level and two sides of the lower level. All of these windows were smashed, the shattered glass spread over the carpeted floor and glue spread over that. Every electrical outlet and every switch was smashed with a heavy pipe. Toilets and sinks were demolished on both levels. It was a sickening sight.

Marian, Lynn and our two young grandchildren, accompanied by Judy Salzman, a church camp counselor, had gone to our all-but-completed Colorado home, expecting to spend a week there. Instead, they discovered the vandals' handiwork.

Peter, our older son, was then living in Silver Plume, Colorado, a few miles west of Georgetown, but he didn't have a phone. When Judy called me to find out what they should do next, I suggested they go to Idaho Springs and try to get a room at the Indian Springs Motel while I tried to get in touch with Pete.

Long distance operators were very helpful, as was the proprietor of the Silver Plume Saloon, who located Pete and let him know his father wanted him to take care of his mother, sister and his sister's two children, stranded at the Albrecht's Colorado homestead. I left instructions for Peter to call me as soon as he arrived at the vandalized house and had assessed the situation.

A radiologist friend, Dr. Bill Claybaugh, arranged to take me out to Colorado in his private plane the next day. A sudden storm came up after we refueled in Lincoln, Nebraska, and gave us quite a scare. Thunder and lightning surrounded us, and the plane gave us the impression of being a roller coaster ride.

This storm forced us one hundred and fifty miles south of our original destination, but we got there only a few hours late, just a little worse for wear.

So often seeming catastrophes turn out to be blessings in disguise. Pete, who had been badly wounded in Vietnam while we vacationed in Mexico in 1969, had lost contact with his family. This incident re-established a good family relationship between us that endures to this day.

Peter supervised repairs, fell in love with the house and eventually bought it from us at a bargain. After several years, he sold it to move closer to his work and now lives in Idaho Springs, Colorado.

A poignant memory is of reading of Peter's wounds in a letter from a black soldier friend of his, long before we were officially notified he was injured. We actually had to telephone our representative in Washington, Congressman Steiger, and then Secretary of Defense Melvin Laird, who was originally from Wisconsin and a personal friend of my uncle Marvin Keil. Both of these individuals had their staffs work over a weekend to get information about Peter's condition to us.

The following Monday morning, we were contacted by the Red Cross. We found out he was to be flown to Colorado.

Marian and I flew to Denver, but wasted four days waiting for Pete to arrive at Fitzsimmons Air Force Base. Frantic calls failed to disclose his whereabouts, other than that his plane had left the West Coast.

I returned home, leaving Marian in Denver. A day later, I had a call from Pete. He was in Illinois! The plane carrying him and several other wounded soldiers had the misfortune of being taken over by top Army brass who insisted on being flown hither and yon, to points of their preference rather than taking the wounded soldiers directly to Fitzsimmons as planned!

Both Pete and I got in touch with Marian and let her know when the plane was to land in Colorado.

Pete, who had lost about eighty pounds, insisted on getting on his feet to meet his mother. While he had lost a third of his bowel, had a hernia and a paralyzed right leg from a shrapnel injury to the femoral nerve, he told her not to worry, he would be skiing again that winter. And, indeed, he did! Pete also taught other wounded soldiers how to ski using a short ski on his right leg.

By the time of the vandalism of our house, Peter had recovered enough to be able to make a living at hard physical work. Truly, God does work in mysterious ways to shape our lives.

While I think all of our children have been scarred by my years of being a practicing workaholic, in retrospect, considering the terrible shortage of physicians in the '50s and '60s, there was little I would do differently. I am grateful that Marian put up with my eccentricities and compulsions, careful to make the most of a bad situation.

CHAPTER

26

"National Day
of Prayer"

W hile driving to a home call one day in April
1970, I happened to have my car radio on at
the time when President Nixon eulogized a recently deceased,
long-time member of the White House Press Corps. Then, as
now, our nation was faced with many problems and divisions.
The thought occurred to me that some years earlier, when
Dwight Eisenhower was president, there had been a National
Day of Prayer. Wouldn't it be wonderful, I thought, if we as a
nation could unite under God's guidance, with the religious leaders of the day leading the nation in prayer? Perhaps this could
be led by Rev. Billy Graham, I thought. And all radio and TV
networks could be mobilized, directing their attention to a prayer
session at our nation's capitol.

The following Sunday, as I greeted my adult Sunday School

class after opening prayer, I mentioned my vision before introducing the planned subject of the day. After a few moments of discussion, the class was unanimous in encouraging me to go ahead. We went back into prayer session and asked God's guidance on how to go about making it happen.

Pastor Morris Wee, who had been so influential in shaping my life in my earlier years at Madison, was now senior pastor at Central Lutheran Church in Minneapolis. With bated breath and with my Sunday school students praying, I used the church phone to ask for information and was pleased, but not really surprised, to catch Morrie between one of his four services that Sunday. I told him of my vision and asked if he had any suggestions on how to go about getting it done.

He suggested I call Bishop Schiotz of the American Lutheran Church, and James M. Johnson, religion editor of the *Milwaukee Sentinel* for advice. Morrie indicated that turning my vision into reality would be a formidable challenge. He wished me well and would pray that if it would be in accordance with God's will, my idea for a revival of the National Day of Prayer would be successful.

We did get through to the bishop that same day, with the same message. In the remaining ten or fifteen minutes of class time, we brainstormed on how to go about this project. We decided that its only hope would be an ecumenical effort directed to all of God's people, starting with all the denominations in our own area, asking the pastors, priests and lay people for suggestions and help. By this time, our pastor, Gerald Monge, had joined our group discussion. We all sensed the presence of God as we joined in the Lord's Prayer following our petition for guidance.

Lloyd Larson, then sports editor at the *Milwaukee Sentinel* newspaper, and James R. Johnson, helped immeasurably with their advice and knowledge of who to contact.

Miracles do occur! The ensuing interdenominational outpouring of support was gratifying. Almost every denomination in the West Bend area willingly responded with help from both clergy and lay people. A one-time donation of one thousand dollars to Christ Lutheran Church financed the whole venture. The passage of time has erased from my mind which of God's children came up with the methods we used to enable us to personally address five thousand letters to all members of the House of Representatives, Senate, Supreme Court, all television station managers, daily newspapers with circulations of over twenty-five thousand in the United States, as well as executive officers of the thousand largest corporations in the United States. Journals, weekly and monthly magazines and denominational and interdenominational organizations were all covered. In the May 23, 1970 *Milwaukee Sentinel* there was an article headed "ALC Backs Prayer Day."

It was a thrilling day at Jackson's Christ Lutheran Church Fellowship Hall when many willing hands addressed copies of my May 15 letter to President Nixon. The letter was accompanied by a cover letter written by Reverend Monge, dated May 29, and clippings of various newspaper articles — including a May 16 *News of Religion* article by James M. Johnson.

This was probably the largest mailing the Jackson Post Office ever had. It went out on the wings of many prayers, resulting in a proclamation by President Nixon on September 15 designating October 21 the National Day of Prayer.

My vision for the National Day of Prayer ultimately did not fully materialize as I had first seen it, but a seeming miracle did happen!

While the proclamation was made on September 25, I did not receive word of it until October 18 via a telephone call from reporters of the *Milwaukee Journal* and *Milwaukee Sentinel*. They called me while I was in Des Moines, Iowa, just before I was to participate in an evangelism rally at Highland Park Lutheran Church.

The previous August, the resource person at our Way Post Church Camp, Reverend Charlie Schmitz, suggested that I consider participating in a new program of evangelism for the American Lutheran Church. While Marian thought it an odd offer, one that was trying to make a "silk purse out of a sow's ear," I accepted the challenge. I had an exciting experience at a preliminary conference in Minneapolis, and a three day rally at Trinity Lutheran Church in Arlington, South Dakota, followed by the October 16, 17, and 18 rally at Highland Park Lutheran Church in Des Moines. We discussed "Drugs and the Devil," "Sex, Sin and Society," "The Generation Gap," and "A New Approach To Stewardship" at the three-day rally.

Only one of my sermons for the rally has survived the passage of time, my contribution to the generation gap discussion, entitled "Giving and Getting."

As mentioned, I have been blessed over the years with an efficient and dedicated office staff. Among their contributions, are several extensive files which I thought had not survived the 1983 merger of the Jackson Medical Service Corporation and the General Clinic. A long-time friend and former employee, Sue Calhoun, surprised me as I was lamenting how was I ever going to remember, with accuracy, all of the things I wanted to include in this account of my life. In response, Sue, who currently assists me part time in keeping my record, presented me with several more files related to the National Day of Prayer.

The joy of having the lost found was tempered with the concern that no book could possibly contain all the materials now available. At the risk of omitting something important, I have abstracted some of the more pertinent material relating to the National Day of Prayer in this book.

CHAPTER

27

"Historical Perspectives"

(Parts of this chapter were
developed from
The History of Jackson — 1843 to 1976)

In the mid-1970s, as part of an effort by the Wisconsin Academy of Family Practice to stimulate interest in family practice among future doctors, a series of medical students worked with me for eight to ten weeks during the summers between the students' first and second years in medical school. This program was held in conjunction with the University of Wisconsin Medical School and the Medical College of Wisconsin in Milwaukee. There was usually only one student, but sometimes I had two.

With the help of colleagues at the hospital and other offices, we were able to keep the students busy. At that time, I spent six years as clinical director of the then new Mental Health Unit of Washington County, and one tumultuous year as medical director of the county's Samaritan Nursing Home, so it was not difficult for me to arrange work for my visiting medical students.

It was my philosophy that doctors should be aware of what other members of the health team contribute. So, my students were assigned to work with the nurses and aides on the night shift alternate weeks, learning to empty bedpans, insert catheters, and comfort the dying and their relatives. In addition to these responsibilities, a student with this assignment had to prepare a list of patients I was to see at six the next morning and become acquainted with the reasons the nurses wanted me to see those particular patients. The student had to be prepared to give me a thumbnail sketch of the physical, mental and emotional problems involved, together with suggestions on what laboratory work should be ordered.

The student who was to work with me during the day started at 6 a.m. at the Samaritan Nursing Home or the Mental Health Unit, which were in the same building, and then stay with me for hospital rounds, office work and night call. The student who had worked all night would stay with me through the hospital rounds or assist with surgery and be excused to rest for the next stint of duty at eleven o'clock that evening.

One of my students, Gary Herdrich, impressed me with his workaholic tendencies similar to mine. We were mutually agreeable to continuing our relationship. I asked him to join my Jackson Medical Service, Inc.

Before Dr. Herdrich finished his residency, the General Clinic purchased a plot of land in Jackson and told me they planned to build a branch medical facility there, hiring two doctors who would be starting about the time Gary was to join me.

Gary was alarmed. He was concerned about what would happen if, after he joined my practice, I would die or be forced for some reason to leave my practice. He then would have to face the competition from two doctors alone. So arrangements were made, despite the apprehension of John Miller, my professional management counselor, to add two new doctors to my practice instead of one.

Dr. Sandy Byerly was in the same residency training program as Gary, at St. Michael's Hospital in Milwaukee. I met Sandy in October and I invited her to join us at the completion of her residency.

I arranged for my soon-to-be-new-associates to be my guests at a County Medical Society meeting and informed the physicians there of my plans. At about the same time, I introduced Dr. Herdrich and Dr. Byerly at a dinner party for the Jackson Business Association, of which I was a charter member. I started publicizing the fact that Jackson would be having two new young family physicians in addition to the supplemental, part-time services provided by physicians from the Parkview Clinic in Hartford and Dr. M.Y. Kahn, a surgeon. All of these people were very kind in helping me hold my practice together while I waited for Dr. Herdrich and Dr. Byerly to complete their residencies. Additional help from the Frankow-Grundahl Clinic in West Bend, sharing the service of their two new family practice associates, Dr. Larry Gill and Dr. Bruce Griswold, in the year before Gary and Sandy joined me was also mutually advantageous.

The association with Dr. Herdrich and Dr. Byerly enabled me to resume my hobby of throwing pots, which I had briefly enjoyed in the mid-1960s, when Marian took an interest in ceramics. In trying to protect me from my work, she encouraged me to join her in her ceramics hobby. When I countered that I would do it if I could get to be a real potter, she arranged for her ceramics instructor, Dorothy Zuber of West Bend, and a retired police officer, who was an experienced potter, to teach me the potter's wheel, one night a week.

As usual my impulsive nature got the better of me. I bought a belt-driven potter's wheel and installed it on a twelve-foot canvas in the middle of the family room in the lower level of our home. The canvas protected the floor while the wheel was in operation. However, whenever the telephone would ring four or five times while I was throwing a pot, the adjacent floor, stairway and telephone, as well as the wall where the telephone was located, would become a clay-encrusted mess.

By mutual consent, that phase of my career was interrupted for the next fifteen years, until Drs. Gill and Griswold made it possible for me to resume my hobby. The five months I have been working on this book is the longest period since 1981 that I have been away from the wheel.

28

"A Trip Back to My Roots"

On January 16, 1993, I awoke with the realization that I was homesick for the places I had enjoyed in my youth so long ago. I had breakfast at six o'clock and called my daughter Lynn about 6:20 a.m. to tell her I was going back home to Beaver Dam, where the story of my life started.

During the last five or six years of her life, my mother always anticipated visits on alternate weekends by Marian and me and my sister Marge and her husband Bill. But since my mother's death in July 1988 we were able to visit the area on only one or two occasions, even though the distance was only about forty miles.

The probable impetus for my decision that "today was the day" to return to Beaver Dam, was a phone call I made to the

First National Valley Bank, formerly the Old National Bank, in Beaver Dam. I was informed that Tom Fisher, who I mentioned earlier was president of the bank, had retired a year ago. Various friends had read in the *Beaver Dam Daily Citizen* of Marian's death and had sent their condolences. Thus, the call to my daughter that I was going to visit boyhood haunts and friends.

Nostalgia is a powerful emotion. While the topography may be the same, changes over the seventy years of my memory are astronomical. When I wrote the "History of Medicine in Jackson" in 1976 for a community historical record, I estimated that perhaps one percent of the people in the area were farmers while the rest had more urban-oriented occupations. Now, less than one in five thousand of the people we see are actively farming.

As dawn was breaking that January morning, with the hoarfrost on the trees and shrubs, I saw the lights indicating chores and milking going on in only four of the farms I passed on the drive from my home to West Bend, a distance of eight miles. The entire thirty-six miles from West Bend to Beaver Dam, I only saw six lighted barns, denoting activity comparable to the days I milked cows. In the early morning light, many boarded up barns and abandoned remains of barns, as well as chicken houses and hog houses and vacant windows decryed the passage of time and the change of an entire way of life during the life spans of the last two generations. Many people still live in the old farm houses, but few families have been able to survive financially running a one-family farm without the husband, wife or children working off the farm to supplement the family's income.

I would expect that none of the five closed cheese factories I saw that early morning drive — one on County Highway A where I used to deliver milk by buggy when staying at Uncle Walde's farm, or at the intersection of County Highway A and

State Highway 151 at the Buckhorn Corners Cheese Factory where I delivered milk when I was helping Uncle Art Heuer — today have anything like the appearance they had when they were functioning cheese factories.

Uncle Art's farm has long since been demolished and has become a waste disposal site for the byproducts from the near-by Green Giant Canning Company. The beautiful trees are gone.

The farms in the Beaver Dam area are probably a little more functional as farms than those around Jackson. But one has to drive another thirty miles to see a preponderance of family farms.

On County Highway B, along the route our threshing and silo-filling crews took to the farms we worked in the '30s and '40s, only one farm that is still actively farming has any semblance to its remembered appearance. Uncle Herb Butterbrodt's house and barn on County Highway A was the only set of farm buildings kept in good shape by apparently loving new owners that I saw while driving around my old haunts.

As dawn broke, I stopped at the old Maple Hill Farm where I was born. There no longer were any maples present. The barn and silo had long since been removed. The twenty acres lost during the Depression are now filled with homes, and I believe there is an extra row of homes on another ten or twenty acres of former farmland. The old sink holes and ponds have been filled in. The orchard and pine trees are long gone.

The old house was torn down when Harry and his wife Betty lived there. The old windmill, laundry and woodshed are gone. Only two of the buildings Harry had built and one of the hog barns remain. The barnyard, berry patch, fences and roads have all been altered.

I am grateful to the young boy who answered the doorbell and gave me permission to walk around the property. I only stayed ten or fifteen minutes and did not walk down to the back forty as I had planned. Whether I will ever get up the courage to explore further, to see if the raspberry bushes or their descendants, are still there is debatable.

The old red brick Jefferson School of Joint District No. 2 still stands, converted into a home. The outside pump and outhouse are no longer there. The evergreen and maple trees are largely gone.

Art Keyser's home is pretty much as I remember it from twenty or twenty-five years ago, but it looks different than it did in 1927 when I listened to the arrival of Lindberg in Paris and the Dempsey-Tunney fight on Art's Atwater-Kent radio. The barn and sheds have long since been removed. The modern home on the other side of County Highway B, built many years ago by his son Merlin and his wife, had a light on. So I stopped and had a very enjoyable visit recalling old times.

Following that, I proceeded east and mourned the sorry condition and dramatic changes to my uncle Walde's and Grandma and Grandpa Albrecht's farm where I had, for so many years, enjoyed farm life in a less competitive era. You can take the boy off the farm, but you can't take the farm out of the boy.

Bernie Maas, living southeast of Charlie Bachhofen's cheese factory, still lives in his modern farm house, but he sold his surrounding farmland. We had a short, but pleasant, visit.

My next stop was a visit to Tom and Carla Faber, next door neighbors and friends of my mother for many years after she moved to Beaver Dam. They indicated the people who had bought the home my mother had shared with my stepfather Brady Cain were an energetic young couple with three children. The young mother reminded the Fabers how energetic my mother had been in her younger years. Tom and Carla were happy to show me a picture Marian had painted of the beautiful trees and homes on the street where they lived, which they inherited when mother died.

My next stop was the office of the First Evangelical Lutheran Church to leave a copy of "Into Life Eternal," which I had written on the night of Marian's death. I spoke to Pastor Russell Miller on the phone, who informed me that Pastor Harold Kuester, who had been semiretired at the time of mother's death, was still active. Pastor Kuester conducted the funeral service at my request. I also discussed the possibility of coming to the old home church sometime next summer to allow my old friends in Beaver Dam to have the opportunity to see the prints of Marian's paintings and my autobiography.

I then enjoyed a visit with Tom Fisher and his wife and let him know I was sorry I wouldn't be able to personally hand him the last payment on the mortgage he helped me arrange. He was glad to know that even though he had taken an early retirement I would be justifying the faith he and Howard Schoenwetter, his predecessor, had in me so many years ago.

The Fisher's were able to tell me where Howard's wife Marie lived — just a few houses from theirs. They were also able to provide the address for Jessie Belle Keller, the widow of my old friend, Dr. Edward Keller, who taught me so much about osteopathy, philosophy and religion. Tom and his wife, as well as Marie Schoenwetter, remembered having been at our silver wedding anniversary at the Linden Inn, a restaurant and banquet facility on Big Cedar Lake, a few miles southwest of West Bend.

Marie had not been home when I called her earlier in the morning, but she was home when I left the Fisher's. We had an enjoyable visit with memories of the letter I had exchanged with her ten years earlier when Howard had died and been buried without my knowing about it until some months later, when I visited Tom at the bank. We stayed in touch since then with an occasional Christmas card, and she sent me a copy of Marian's obituary from the *Beaver Dam Daily Citizen* with a note of condolence. We had a mutually agreeable visit.

My next stop was for a belated lunch at the Country Kitchen, a restaurant we often had taken my mother and her companion to during the last four or five years of Mother's life. Doreen Koch, a friend, had stayed with mother after Brady died.

After lunch, one of the waitresses was able to direct me to the Beaver Dam Care Center where Jessie Belle Keller had been an active volunteer and resident since shortly after my last visit to Beaver Dam, at the time of my mother's death. We picked up the threads of our friendship much more easily than anyone would imagine, bringing each other up-to-date on friends and relatives.

The trip home was uneventful, except for the ability to see many cash crops — fields of corn still unharvested — deeply embedded in snow. While farming has drastically changed over the course of my lifetime, one thing is as true now as it has always been over the years. Humankind can do little to change the weather patterns ordained by God.

CHAPTER

29

"Body, Mind and Spirit"

Just as I had despaired to recall any meaningful experiences of the mid-'70s, and after a several day hiatus in dictating, another miracle happened. A friend and patient since February 11, 1976, Christof H. Mittmann, was in my office for a routine appointment, a recheck of a recurrent lower back sprain treated a month earlier. While Chris is twenty-two years younger than I, I have always empathized with his problem. Like me, he has had trouble with his back since an early age. In his case, since he was five or six, whereas my problem didn't start until I was thirteen.

During the course of treatment, when I told him I was writing an autobiography, he asked if he was going to be in it, and asked if he could have an autographed copy when it was completed.

During our conversation, we had mentioned the slippery roads and ice of the morning before, which reminded both of us of the great ice storm that hit our area of the country in March 1976. Many homes were without electricity from ten to fourteen days because of that storm. That led to mutual remembrances of one of the more remarkable physician-patient relationships in all my years of practice.

Chris asked if I remembered what I told him when I discharged him from the hospital on March 17, 1976.

When I confessed that I remembered the hospitalization but not what I told him, he said, with tears in his eyes, "When I was thanking you for pulling me through, you told me 'Don't thank me, thank God. I am just a tool.'" We both had some recall of the horrible events relating to his hospitalization during the ice storm, when ice caused electric wires and poles to collapse in the area surrounding the hospital, amid loud cracking sounds and electric blue flashes.

While initially I had planned on identifying by name only a few patients, in the interest of preserving confidentiality, Chris gave his permission for me to abstract and reproduce those portions of his hospital record which not only illustrate the inner relationship of body, mind and spirit, but also illustrate the need for physicians to touch all bases rather than concentrate on only the physical symptoms bringing the patient to the office or hospital. Assembly line medicine, increasingly encouraged by the social planners, with emphasis on cost control, can't help but reduce the pleasures of the practice of medicine. The close, interpersonal relationships between patients and physician now are part of a rapidly vanishing era.

Chris, as a young boy in Germany during World War II, was run over by a beer wagon during an air raid. For the rest of the war he would be strapped to an ironing board and carried to a basement shelter during the air raids that demolished his city.

More than thirty years later, Chris was hospitalized for back pain, in traction one night during the ice storm. The detailed hospital records, including those of Dr. Donald Muth, an internist, on March 6, will be of interest, as well as a history and physical I dictated, unaccustomedly late for me, on March 11. A discharge summary dated March 18 details the events of Chris' two weeks in the hospital.

The hospital progress notes are too extensive to reproduce here. Briefly, Chris was admitted with back pain and put in traction, starting with sixteen pounds and increased in two-pound increments to twenty-six pounds. He was seen in consultation the morning after admission by Dr. Michael Reineck, an orthopedic surgeon, who, that same day, decreased the traction to fifteen pounds. Dr. Reineck felt at the time that the problem appeared to be a strained latisimus dorsi muscle on the right side of Chris' back.

The next day, when Dr. Reineck saw him, Chris was having pain and numbness in his right hand, elbow and the right side of his ribs. Valium was substituted for Soma, a muscle relaxant, to see if it would make any difference. By the time I saw Chris at 5:30 the evening of March 5, the spasms were less intense and the arm was better, but Chris thought that was from the Ronniacal, given to relieve muscle spasms in arterial walls, started during the day. Dr. Reineck also had ordered five milligrams of Valium to be administered orally with Chris' meals and 10 milligrams at night.

Dr. Reineck's note earlier on March 6 indicated the "patient [was] more comfortable in traction; the pain in the right arm ... may need a nerve conduction study. He was complaining of crepitation [repeated crackling sounds] over the lateral rib margin; otherwise stable."

At 12:30 p.m., my dictated entry about the emergency call from the hospital reads, "While eating lunch in presence of [his] wife, severe, sudden pain left anterior thorax [chest], shortness of breath, confusion and apprehension. Kept speaking, 'liver, liver.' [He] was eating liver at the time, but there was no evidence of aspiration. Denied radiation of the pain on the right. Pulse was regular at 120. Chest clear. Respirations 32. Blood Pressure 140/120–100. Power [of his grasp] was good."

My impression was "probably pulmonary embolus; doesn't appear to be conversion hysteria; patient in some respects gives that impression."

Chris had been given two Empirin No. 3, a pain reliever containing aspirin and codeine, before his meal and had no problem with these before. His hands and feet were sweaty and his body was warm. An arterial blood gas study was started.

Dr. Muth was consulted. Chris was moved to intensive care and seen at 2:30 and 4:30 that afternoon. At 5 p.m. he was more comfortable.

Chris remained critical at 7:30 a.m. on March 7. A lung scan was ordered, but it was not very helpful. Chest x-rays taken at the time probably showed a slight increase in the size of Chris' heart when compared to the day before, but that, too, did not shed much light on the source of his problem. His heart sounds were too good for us to be seriously thinking of pericarditis or effusion. Eye motion during a funduscopic exam made it difficult to exclude cerebral edema as a possible culprit.

I visited Chris at 2:45 p.m. March 7. That visit shed a lot of light on the case.

The attending nurse, who was with Chris the day before and before his acute pain began, mentioned that during the previous morning, Chris had been very talkative. He spoke of the similarity of the loud cracking and flashes of light when a power line hit the ground outside the hospital the night before to his experiences in Germany during the war. As a boy, Chris had been pressed into service as an ammunition carrier. The sudden cracking sounds and the flashing lights of the ice-shattered electric power poles reactivated long-suppressed, subconscious fears experienced during the war of his childhood.

That night in the hospital, Chris tried to reach for his shoes so he could leave his room, and it frightened him to be tied down to the bed in traction. Subconsciously, he was reminded of the terror he experienced during the war, when he was tied to the ironing board to be carried down into the air raid shelter.

I had a conference with his sister and wife. (I believe this was before I learned of Dr. Charles Whittaker, who advocated consulting with the family and the patient together when working with emotional problems. He taught a postgraduate course I attended in the same general period.)

The conference with his sister and wife confirmed Chris' hardship as a boy during the war. His sister stated Chris probably had the roughest childhood of the three siblings. His father had been killed in 1940, when Chris was two-and-one-half years old, and his mother had been a dominating figure in his life. The family's home at one time had been demolished in a windstorm.

Chris had been sickly as an infant, his sister said, and according to his mother, supposedly had a hole between the upper chambers of the heart. His sister was not aware of any tests being done on his heart, because the family had lived in a tiny village. At the age of six, weighing only twenty-six pounds, Chris had a stomach problem and vomiting. This accompanied his hardships during the war.

About the same period he had been run over by the beer truck and was told he would never walk again because of the back injury. He also had told his wife he had artificial kneecap implants, the knee injuries apparently also caused by the beer truck.

Early in 1945, at the age of seven, he was shot in the right elbow by a strafing airplane while he, his sister and a couple of other children were playing in a field. At another time,

Chris had run home from school without his clothing, frightened by an air raid.

In 1945, right before a German general was captured by American troops in Bavaria, the general hid his handgun in Chris' pocket. Later, when she discovered the gun, Chris' mother took him to the family's outhouse where she threw the gun away.

Chris had also been brought up to be fearful of thunderstorms and taught to get up and light a candle whenever one occurred.

He had gone through the February 13, 1945 night-long firebombing of Dresden; remembering the bodies, flames and smells.

Chris had been placed in a German orphanage for a while in 1948, when the family was having financial difficulty. He had a nervous breakdown while in the orphanage. There had been no known psychiatric care, yet Chris had told his sister about a year earlier that he didn't have long for this world.

When he was older, Chris was pushed to be the head of the family. Chris later told his wife and sister that he wished his mother had not refused to move the family into a refugee camp after the war. Instead, she collected her two sons and one daughter and came to this country in 1956.

Chris' sister had talked with him for about an hour a month before his hospitalization when they discussed his mother having sent him a hate letter, remonstrating against his marrying outside the Catholic faith.

Unfortunately, in the '60s and '70s, many Protestants and Catholics had greater allegiance to their denominations than to God. Even with his ingrained training, along with his adherence to the Fourth Commandment, Chris found it impossible to honor his mother's wishes, and impossible to obey her in the matter of his marriage. This had a great effect on him.

He had worked at a well-paying job, his sister said, but progressively in the last few months, as the work force was reduced, a portion of the business having been sold, he worried that his job would collapse under him.

Chris was afraid to look for another job because he had never learned to spell in American English, though he could read well. He understood English words and could print words, but he was unable to translate his German thoughts into written American words. Chris went through the eighth grade plus three years of apprenticeship and business administration in Germany. He has been a machinist since 1956 and was a plant manager at the time of his hospitalization, but without the authority he felt he should have.

It was my impression that Chris' condition was probably a combination of physical and emotional factors, and that it was quite possible both were being compounded by the other.

Chris did instruct his wife before she left the hospital the day before what to do when he died. He had been joking with her about death for the past month or so and had told his sister he had a weak heart.

The progress note of the next day indicated Chris was feeling and looking better. On March 8, he answered the question mentioned earlier about his saying "liver, liver." He explained that indeed a piece of liver momentarily caught in his throat, but it later came out.

Subsequent notes over the next ten days showed progressive improvement in all respects until his discharge on March 17, 1976.

Those killed in war are but a tiny portion of the human casualties. The lives of all are scarred by the inhumanity of man against man. I often wonder how much longer God can continue to have patience with the imperfect people he originally created in His image.

While the time of judgement comes to each of us as individuals, it seems to me very likely the judgement of God will ultimately result in the fall of our civilization, even as civilizations of the past have failed to survive the consequences of reliance on self rather than God. Civilization's obsession with treasures on earth ultimately will reduce the enjoyment of life both here and in the hereafter.

30

"Modern Farming — Trip to the Kratz Farm"

I made a trip to visit Richard Kratz and his farms one day in January. Richard is a long-time friend and patient of mine who lives near Jackson.

Many times during his routine physical examinations, we would end up talking about his farms. He would describe the many automated marvels found on a modern farm and I would describe how we ran a farm fifty years ago.

Richard invited me to visit his farming operation, and I finally took him up on the offer, wanting to see for myself how much farming has changed in the past half century.

The Kratz's main home farm of three hundred acres as well as a nearby farm of one hundred and seventy-seven acres are operated by the three Kratz brothers, Richard, James and Gary, and their brother-in-law Allen Emmer. A few years ago, these four formed a partnership and bought a one hundred and eighty-acre farm without buildings near Iron Ridge in Dodge County. The remainder of the 1,805 acres they farm is leased. Having their cropland so widely dispersed provides a safety mechanism against local climactic catastrophes.

The partners own their equipment and livestock. Each of the four partners has his own area of expertise and responsibility. Majority rules when there is a difference of opinion.

In his home, Richard showed me a picture of the farm taken in 1965, which corresponds pretty much with the time I remember my brother caring for our home farm and four additional farms he rented.

Since then, the Kratz farm house on the north side of Sherman Road has been remodeled. The farm buildings remaining from the era of the photo include a forty-by-sixty-foot machine shed, which is pretty much unchanged. One silo from that time also is unchanged. The shed just south of the silo remains, as does the main barn, although both have been extensively added to and remodeled. What was a barn cleaner shed then, at the end of the main barn, is now a calf shed. The open-fronted building to the north in the photo, called the "loafing" barn for the cows, burned down in 1968 and was replaced with a long and narrow, free-stall barn, shown in a another photograph taken in 1979.

As Richard recalls, that barn was put up in 1968 to replace the burned one. In the 1979 photo, there are five silos, a long feeder in the yard around which numerous cows are gathered, two farm yards adjacent to each other separated by a fence, and a manure storage tank, which had been installed in 1977. The comparison with the photo of twelve years earlier shows further astronomical changes. In the later picture, there are four buildings that did not appear on either of the others. The yard, which had been divided into four areas, has been replaced by one of the new buildings. There are now two smaller yards between the main building and the manure storage area called a slurry. Pasture and crop areas have been changed. The various areas have different equipment, which is no longer used only a few years later. *Tempes fuget.*

A few steps to his desk and Richard showed me a computer, which has details of all of the farms he operates, field by field, section by section — farming details never thought of in the era of my recollection. I remember his telling me about the computer, which he dreamed of getting about three years ago. He actually got the computer two years ago and taught himself how to use it. Richard has developed books for all seven of his fellow workers detailing each farm field, crops for all the 1,805 acres worked, size to the tenth of an acre, and the input going into each one. This enables each of their employees to know exactly what is going on day to day, and to have an accurate perception of the productivity of each area of the field, which will help them next season in knowing what fertilizers to use and where to distribute it.

Richard said that in the near future, satellite photography will provide even more information to farmers.

I found it almost impossible to believe that one person could absorb that much knowledge, but Richard indicated that he goes to seminars and keeps himself up-to-date. In fact, only days before I had stopped in he was at such a seminar, learning more about fertilizer and pesticides.

We drove to the main farm where the buildings, which looked large on the picture, seem even more huge when standing next to them. In the milk house, there was a stainless steel container, which can hold up to one thousand five hundred gallons of milk. On an adjacent wall is a milk slip recording that the weight shipped the day before was 9,746 pounds. That morning, 9,660 pounds of milk were shipped. Earlier in the month, 9,916 pounds were shipped one day. The fluctuation resulted from the number of cows being milked and perhaps on the weather. Cows are sometimes switched from one place to another, and sometimes production declines are due more to fewer cows available for milking than on less production per cow.

We then went to the milking parlor where on either side of a central, recessed alleyway there are eight milking machines. The cows enter eight at a time on either side of the recessed alleyway, guided by an occasional mild electric shock from a fence if they stray too far off the proper path. The door to the milking parlor is opened automatically when a button is pushed. In fact, all operations are automatic, with the electricity provided by one of several backup generators on the farms in case of a catastrophe.

I asked Richard how long it would take to get their generators working in the event of another ice storm like we experienced in 1976. With no emergency generators at that time, he said the farm was without electricity for two weeks after the storm. They installed the generators, which now can put them back into operation in five minutes. These generators are run by gasoline engines, not by a tractor as I visualized. They do have seven or eight tractors on their different farms.

The only thing done by hand, as I recall, is the actually placing the milking machine's four tit-cups on the cows; they come off automatically. Each udder and tit is wiped off with a damp towel prior to application of the tit cups. In an adjacent room is another computer which records the daily production of each cow, the status of the cow as to total production, dates when the cow was bred or should be bred, and dates when the cow was dry. The computer also automatically determines which cows are not profitable.

Any one of the four partners in the farm is able to access this information. On one recent day, there was a total production of 9,166 pounds from one hundred and seventy-nine cows. That averaged out to 54.8 pounds per cow for the day. The farm's overall average was 55.6. Average time for each milking was 7.4 minutes.

I think the only statistic they don't have is the amount of manure production per cow!

As I went through a narrow metal gate, I was told that the computer identifies each cow by reading its metal tag as the cow passes. I didn't have the appropriate tag, so the computer did not acknowledge me.

The next stop on my tour was an adventure in the free-stall barn, which holds two hundred head. It had a concrete floor with a corrugated surface to prevent the cows from slipping. There were three different areas into which the cows are separated for production. In each area there is a raised platform on which they can eat, sleep and drink. The floor, itself, is cleaned twice a day of excrement by a skidloader that pushes the manure into a collection pit under the floor. This pit holds one hundred fifty thousand gallons when full. The collection pit is emptied about every two weeks, either into an outdoor holding tank or directly into a manure spreader. The manure spreader is entirely unlike those I remember. It is a tank truck that sprays the liquid slurry onto the appropriate fields. When the field is close to a residential area, where people object to the odor, the slurry is injected under the surface of the soil to cut down on the smell.

The feeding for the cows is arranged by computer according to the individual cow's production. Top producers get a higher and richer amount of the formula.

Our next stop was the heifer shed, containing thirty-five or forty heifers. Each heifer is labeled with an ear piece showing the date of birth and the father's name. Some have numbered codes. Breeding has long since become an entirely artificial procedure in the last thirty years, differing radically from my recollection of leading the cow down to a "scrub bull" on the neighbor's farm.

Outside the barn, perhaps fifty steers are being fed, apparently in that feeding area because the yard was being cleaned.

Next, I learned the difference between Harvestore silos, those big blue silos found on many farms these days, and uprights.

The Harvestore delivers "first in" silage "out first." There is never any old feed. The concrete upright silo, which is almost as large as the Harvestore, with a metal dome, is unloaded from the top down automatically, not with a silage fork, which I was used to in 1930. Adjacent to one of the Harvestore silos is a thirty-ton bin for soybean meal, which is also loaded and unloaded automatically.

We traversed a half dozen steps down to the old dairy barn, now used by about one hundred and fifty heifers and steers, separated by age and sex. There are close to six hundred head of cattle on the Kratz farms, but no bulls. Richard's brother, Jim, does the actual breeding of the cows, with sperm procured from six different breeding establishments.

Segregation by sex is now officially practiced in the dairy industry, if not in American society.

In the lower level of the south end of the same barn, dry cows are separated into two separate pens according to the state of their dryness and how close to calving they are. Here, too, the watering and feeding is all automatic.

As I expressed amazement at what I saw, Richard said there are even more modernized farms with automatic flushing devices that clean the floors of the cattle areas four or five times a day. When I wondered what happened to the excess water, he said it is pumped out after the solid material settles and is used over again.

As we walked out, we saw a fifteen-ton, conically-shaped bin which contains roasted soybeans. These soybeans are fed to the most productive cows automatically, regulated by a computer.

My question on what happens to the calves was answered when I was shown the plastic calf bins, standing vacant.

We moved to the farm's one-hundred-and-twenty-by-thirty-foot building which, in the photo, is the one farthest to the north and the newest building they have. The south wall is actually made of canvass, which, in the summer can be raised to allow the sunlight in, supplementing the solar panels which cover the southern portion of the roof. On the north wall there is a six-inch area of separation between the wall and the ceiling for ventilation.

There were probably forty-five to fifty calves in the building. The calves were individually marked with ear tags and wore individual wire feeders around their necks. The barn is supplied with hot and cold running water. The younger calves are gathered in a row near the north wall and are fed by hand with bottles. As they get older, they drink out of pails. When they are sufficiently old enough to not need the bottle or pail any more, they are moved to the south row where there are plastic containers with nipple-like valved tubes. The nipple tubes fools them into thinking they will be drinking milk, when actually they are fed grain. This method of force feeding allows the calves to grow faster.

To illustrate my lack of knowledge of modern farming methods, I asked Richard how they kept the pipes from freezing in the barn. I was told they use a hydrant-like underground watering system, so there are no water-filled pipes above ground when not in use.

After leaving the calf barn, we enter a seventy-by-one-hundred-forty-foot building, which had a ceiling height of sixteen feet. This building is used for warehousing and storage of some of the farm equipment.

Richard got a great deal of enjoyment out of showing me how the twelve-row corn planter could be transported by road from one farm to the next. I wasn't able to grasp his explanation when he told me about it in the office the previous spring. I couldn't really believe that instead of two rows they planted twelve at a time. After seeing the corn planter, I understood how it was possible.

The planter's telescoping mechanism is constructed in such a way that the corn planter spins around on the trailer with the machine's weight completely carried by four wheels in the center. So, by turning at ninety degrees and adjusting a few knobs, it becomes operational. The trailer stays with the planter during operations in the field. The telescoping mechanism is what I hadn't visualized when he told me about it in my office.

The thirty-foot rotary hoe has the same width as the twelve-row planter and replaces the drag and corn cultivator I remember from my youth. It also replaces some of the pesticides used during the era when my brother Harry was running the farms at Beaver Dam, although some pesticide sprays are still needed.

Essentially, I understood the application of fertilizer one inch below and two inches to the side of the corn. The fertilizer is dropped ahead of the corn, with the planter's press wheels trailing behind, closing the furrow. But one of the things I had never even heard of before was a spray bonnet behind the row unit of the planter. This spray bonnet can be automatically controlled to disperse herbicide either in a narrow band of about six inches on either side of the row or, where there are a lot of weeds, over the whole area. This reduces the cost of chemicals and production.

In an earlier chapter, I mentioned how farmers always took pride in being able to produce straight crop rows. Now, with the much more sophisticated tractors available than we had in the '30s and '40s, farmers have a guidance system mounted right on their corn planters. Despite what the the tractor does, the corn planter makes straight rows, which I have admired while driving past farm fields over the last few years.

I also marvelled at the twelve-row corn cultivator, which seems to be an awfully expensive thing to own for the once or twice a year cultivation required these days, compared to the five to six times per season during my farm era.

A bent wire, about three-eighths of an inch in diameter, in a control box, by some pressure mechanism guides the cultivator to go in the right row. Simultaneously, a mechanism called "weed and feed" puts nitrogen and other necessary fertilizer in a given field. It sprays it right next to the roots at the rate of six gallons an acre.

Tanks of two-hundred and fifty gallons, two at a time, are carried on the front of the tractor to supply enough nitrogen or weed spray for about twenty acres. When in operation, these tanks have to be refilled three or four times a day.

Another machine, called a grain vac, replaces the grain bags I used to carry, sucking grain from the bin by a vacuum and simultaneously blowing it onto the truck. *No more shovels* — and ten minutes to load one thousand bushels onto the semi! No more backaches, either! The grain vac also blows the corn up through a metal tube at the top of the Harvestore silo.

As I visualized the Farmall tractor of my later youth, I was shown a two-hundred and thirty-five horsepower marvel with a heated and air-conditioned cab. This modern tractor has eight huge tires, with the side tires separated by about ten or twelve inches, coinciding with the rows of corn they are to avoid.

Even with my relatively stiff knees and back, I was able to ascend three steps and approximately five feet into the cab of this monster. The cab has all the comforts of home, plus a computer that greeted me with a verbal "hello" when I pressed a button. This computer weighs the crops being harvested, through a pipe arrangement attached to a scale. The tractor's tilt steering wheel would give due credit to a Cadillac.

The air-ride seat gave me an understanding why Richard hasn't been in more often to see me to have his back taken care of. Then I thought, after eighteen hours a day of work, typical for a farmer, I didn't know how he would have found time to get over to see me, anyway.

As we were going to see Richard's monstrous combine, we passed a John Deere tractor of vintage I remembered from my brother's farming days back in the '60s. Richard's combine dwarfs the old Farmall I used in the '40s.

While I identified this machine as a combine, as I got into the cab that was perhaps ten or twelve feet above the floor of the equipment shed, I was amazed to see just outside the cab cone-like appendages. I was told these were soybean heads, which are used to harvest wheat and oats, as well as soybeans.

We next went to the building holding the corn heads, which now replace the corn pickers of long ago. These corn heads shell the corn as they go down the field.

This one combine probably replaces at least five men. One man controls this electronic marvel with the on-board computer, which completely regulates the harvesting operation.

One of the most amazing things demonstrated to me was the combine's safety mechanism. I did not quite understand how it worked when Richard explained to me in my office, but on that visit I saw how today's farmers are less likely to lose arms and legs by trying to dislodge stones or other debris from their equipment. There is a hydraulic reverser, avoiding the necessity of the farmer taking a chance on being decapitated while trying to unjam the mechanism.

Another marvelous safety device I could not visualize until my visit was a huge auger, hydraulically lifted up and down to move grain into storage without cranking up the auger. This was seventy feet long.

On the way out of this shed I saw the modern version of the hay tedder, which doesn't resemble anything I remember in the '20s, '30s or '40s when they were still horse drawn.

Into another shed we went, where Richard showed me a

machine he told me about a year or two earlier when I asked whether they still had stone boats to remove rocks from the fields. Richard's machine picks stones over a width of twenty feet with rotating, ten-foot rotors, each with attached six- or eight-inch appendages that push the stones to the center where a reel picks them up and puts them in the bucket to the rear of the machine. This bucket can be picked up and dumped into a truck, eight feet high, to be hauled off the field and dumped. No more rows of stone fences, no more stone boats, and no more back aches!

The next piece of equipment I saw, hard to describe, was mounted on a one-ton pickup truck. It had a computerized control system that regulated the amount of spray delivered from a tank through a boom. It minutely controls the rate of application for whatever they are attempting to put on the field — insecticide or herbicide, for example.

What I considered a new item of equipment when I saw it, is actually obsolete now. It is a forage loading wagon. This has been replaced by a more modern dump box that deposits the grain, after it has been weighed following harvest, into the eighteen-ton trucks that convey the grain to the bins. This machine is painted green and the Kratz's have an equally large red one, used to weigh hay and corn silage before dumping it into a truck. This is on a hydraulic lift which will go up eighteen feet and dump the whole load into the truck. The green grain cart is emptied into the truck with a fourteen-inch auger.

As we left the equipment shed, Richard used a six-row corn picker head to demonstrate how the corn is husked before it goes into the combine, where it is shelled. Stalks and chopped up cobs are expelled back onto the field automatically.

Modern facilities for fuel storage for the present day farmers are regulated by the state's Department of Natural Resources. The Kratz farms have a completely enclosed concrete storage bunker for gasoline and oil, which prevents contamination of the soil and ground water by the petroleum products.

The next shed on my tour sheltered a chisel plow that replaces the moldbar plow and disc I was accustomed to using. In the same shed are plastic tubing and mechanisms used to mix the manure under the surface of the ground. Also stored in this shed are old disc and field cultivators, somewhat similar to what my brother used in the '60s. Another machine, called the pull-by train, was used for incorporating chemicals into the ground in conjunction with herbicides to protect the soybean crops.

The old-fashioned barn, which is not used on many farms anymore, is used on the Kratz farm to store round bales of hay, each weighing about one thousand-five hundred pounds. The barn has an endloader with a grapple fork device that conveys the hay bales and stacks them three tiers high, and can take the bales down and deliver them to the feeding sheds.

Adjacent to this was a pile of soybean straw, which is used for bedding. It seems to be a little coarser than the oat straw I remember using in my youth, but it serves the same purpose.

Before I left that amazing farm, Richard and I visited what will likely be a replacement for the current expensive, state-of-the art, upright modern silos with their substantial maintenance costs. The Kratz's have installed a new ground-level bunker silo. Essentially, it is a concrete platform enclosed by concrete walls twelve to fifteen feet high on three sides. Modern farm trucks can back into this bunker silo and dump their loads of silage; endloaders and other equipment spread the silage evenly and pack it down. When the silo is filled, a plastic sheeting goes over the top to keep the rain out.

Using this storage method, mold should not be as big a factor as it was on the top of the silage in the old silo towers I was used to forty-plus years ago.

The bunker silo seems to incorporate the same principle some farmers of the Depression years used when they dug deep ditches in which they stored their excess silage. While I don't remember personally seeing ditch silos, I remember reading about them as a poor man's alternative to investing money he didn't have for a stave silo, relatively inexpensive though they were then.

At this point, Richard asked if I was up to a side trip to a second farm eight miles away, a relatively recent acquisition by his parents, Robert and Elinor Kratz.

I think he was more amused than surprised at my eager response and we took off for what I considered my visit to a second "transition farm."

On the way we crossed certain roads that I remembered having traveled between Hartford and West Bend in times past when I was seeing patients and giving anesthesia at the hospitals in both cities. I even saw some of the farm homes where I made home calls years ago.

On the way, Richard told me that his parents had acquired much of the family's farmland, which they still own, over the years. As their sons got old enough to take over the farms, Robert went back to his first love, over-the-road truck driving, which he continues to do at age sixty-two.

As I marveled at the complexity of the operation, I reflected on a long-ago visit to a packing plant in Madison where I was told, as we watched the processing of pigs into pork, "The only thing we don't use is the squeal." I asked Richard a question my son Charles once posed, whether the stored manure couldn't be converted to methane gas production. Richard said the idea had been tried a number of years ago, but was not cost effective.

As we drove into the yard of the Kratz's second farm, we saw that even with today's modern equipment, things do not always run as smoothly as planned. Two of the men operating the farm were resignedly chipping away frozen manure from the sides of the spreader. They were still at this unscheduled job about an hour later after we had completed our tour.

Farmers active during my boyhood, youth and middle age would scarcely believe their eyes at the advances made at that farm, which is gradually being brought up to the 1993 standard of the home farm.

There, the cows were still in stanchions. The automatic water dispensers at each cow's head were only a little larger than were those I remember in our old home barn. The odor of the manure and the smell of the cows is about the same. The humidity in the barn is less here than I remembered. The sounds of cows moving around the stanchions were about the same. The automatic feeding mechanism, electronically controlled and computer directed, though not as sophisticated as on the farm we had just left, was enough to amaze me.

A trip to the room under the silo was a revelation. It was entirely dissimilar from the vestibule of the barn of my boyhood from which we carried bushel baskets of silage to put in the mangers for our twenty or so cows and young stock. Back then, the silage had been laboriously thrown out from the top of the silo, after a climb up the iron rungs to the top level. Memory took me back to the sometimes frozen silage attached to the silo walls and made me duplicate in my mind what the farmhands were doing to the frozen manure on the vehicle in the farm's driveway.

It was a little late for Richard to return to the home farm to join in doing the chores. I think I amazed him with my stamina when I expressed my interest in watching the milking operation. I stayed for perhaps another half hour marveling at the precision and automation that was used to milk the cows so efficiently.

I saw first hand how the cows were ushered in, pneumatically locked into place, tags on each cow recording her statistics on an adjacent computer screen. There were sixteen cows, eight on each side of the recessed work area. Every one of those sixty-four tits was cleansed with a germicidal solution using a cup-like device at the top of a plastic bottle. The tits were then dried using recycled toweling. The milking machine tit cups were then put in place. A button was pressed to start the milking operation.

The milk was drawn through plastic tubing into the bucket, automatically weighed and recorded on the computer for that particular cow. That information was compared with the morning production and transmitted electronically to the adjacent room for storage.

It seemed as though each set of sixteen cows was taken care of by one attendant in about twelve or fifteen minutes. During the Depression, when I was hand milking twelve cows an hour, perhaps one-twelfth of today's milk production per cow was considered standard.

Farming has changed considerably since 1850 when John Kratz, Richard's great-great-great-grandfather, homesteaded this farm. Although the equipment used by the family farm has changed over the years, the basic human values have not. The farmer continues to work long, hard hours for low pay. He continues to support America's cheap food policy. Without the farmer, American consumers would be paying a lot more money for the food they purchase. (Americans use one-seventh of each dollar for food. Russians use seventy percent of each dollar for food.)

The family farm would be impossible without the support of the parents who own the land. It would not be a success without the sweat and hard work of their ancestors and the current generation. In the Kratz Family Farm, each generation's sacrifices has made it possible for the present generation to expand and grow. Every farmer is aware his crops would be nothing without the help of our Creator.

As I reflect on what I saw at the Kratz farms, the thought occurred to me that the changes in farming and food production in the past seventy-plus years undoubtedly eclipse the changes that occurred during the preceding 1,916 years. The changes in the healing arts since I was first exposed to them by my relationship with Dr. Keller in 1932 and my entry into the practice of medicine in 1948 are no less dramatic.

31

"Tilting
at
Windmills"

As I reflect on events of this chapter, I am reminded of the question posed during my struggle
with the selective Service in 1940. Augie Butterbrodt, an
esteemed member of our threshing crew, put into words what
most of my friends and acquaintances were thinking. "Are you
really a conscientious objector or just a chronic objector?"

It does seem that he may have been right, as some of my
communications addressed to various levels of government in
1977 and 1978 attest.

* * * * *

November 28, 1977
Mr. Ralph Andreano
Director of Health Policy and Planning
Department of Health and Social Services
State of Wisconsin
Madison, WI 53701

Dear Mr. Andreano:

When you spoke to the Wisconsin Academy of Family Practice at Lake Geneva, you indicated you would welcome questions and suggestions.

Last week, one of my 93-year-old patients, who lives with a daughter, visited me, on 11/22/77. She had previously been seen on 8/17/77, at which time Digoxin, 0.25 mg., 100 [tablets] were prescribed. Because of Medicaid and Medicare rulings, the pharmacist is not permitted to give more than a 30-day supply of any drug. The patient assumed that, because she only had 30 tablets, she didn't need any more and again is in congestive failure.

It has long seemed to me to be ridiculous that an inexpensive drug, such as Digoxin, which once started is almost always continued for the life of the patient, should be limited to a 30-day supply, when the patient needs to be seen only every 2-3-4 months. With many of our patients traveling 10-15 miles or more, it imposes additional costs of transportation as well as inconvenience coming back to the pharmacy every 30 days. The cost of 3 separate prescriptions for 30 tablets each, including the pharmacy fee, is $7.92, while the cost of 100 tablets, filled once, is $3.12.

I am certain that if consideration were given to the realities of this situation, a considerable amount of money could be saved.

Sincerely yours,
James E. Albrecht, MD

March 13, 1978
Department of Health and Social Services
Bureau of Health Care Financing
Room 325, State Office Building
1 W. Wilson Street
Madison, WI 53703

Re: Medicaid "Super-Rule"

On August 6, 1978 I will have been in practice 30 years. During that time I have tried to practice good medicine and render quality care, with adequate documentation of that care, to large numbers of patients. In order to provide that care and documentation, we have found employment of numerous people necessary to enable us to meet the demand for services. Of late years, increased paperwork necessitated by insurance companies, Social Security and Medicaid forms to be filled out, over and above the documentation of patient's care, requires the efforts of 2 people.

Escalating wages and supplies [have] made the allowed fees of Medicare and Medicaid insufficient to cover the costs of care provided. We have a disproportionate number of the disadvantaged in our practice. Unlike some clinics, we have never screened patients on the ability to pay before accepting them as patients. The only restriction we have had in the last few years has been on geographic location of residents in relation to our clinic. We have not tried to screen out the Medicare and Medicaid patients. We are concerned about continuing to provide services at greater costs than we are reimbursed.

Should your proposed policy regarding the authority of reduced payments to physicians in time of budget overruns be passed, the effect would be catastrophic on our practice. Reducing our payroll in order to compensate for such reduction in income would be counter-productive in that it would reduce the number of patients we could adequately care for.

I personally will find it very difficult to even read, much less comprehend, everything in over 300 pages of rules and regulations, which I understand are forthcoming. It would seem quite likely that even the best intentioned and most industrious, intelligent physician will inadvertently be negligent in following such large numbers of rules. Our primary responsibility is to render good care to the patient. Time spent in redundant paperwork, having no relationship to actual care rendered, not only increases costs of operation but detracts from the time available for caring for people.

While we have records detailing our care of all patients since 1948, it does not seem proper to make those records available to anyone, including personnel from your department, without written permission from the patient whose records are to be reviewed. Certainly, private patients would have every right to be indignant if their records were to be reviewed by outsiders, as a part of a comparative study as to how they are treated in comparison with welfare clients.

It seems to me the proposal to make it mandatory for a physician/provider to participate in the continuing medical education program designated by your department is inappropriate and superfluous. Members of the Academy of Family Practice and others have long been keeping current with approved post-graduate educational programs.

Many patients have problems demanding immediate attention, which any physician is obligated to give on a timely basis. Rules should not be made regarding prior authorization to block this timely intervention.

News releases on the amount of reimbursement various physicians throughout the state have received from Medicare and Medicaid seemed to imply wrongdoing on the part of the physicians. It seems to me that many of these men should be given a pat on the back, rather than a kick in the rump, for having the compassion to care for people with yellow cards, whom nobody else wants to care for.

Sincerely yours,
James E. Albrecht, MD

cc: Earl R. Thayer, Secretary
State Medical Society of Wisconsin

* * * * *

March 20, 1978

Governor Martin J. Schreiber
State Capitol
Madison, WI 53702

Dear Governor Schreiber:
I am enclosing a copy of a letter directed on 3/13/78 to the Department of Health and Social Services. Within the last week or two, my office personnel have brought to my attention reimbursement of $3.10 from Wisconsin Medical Assistance, in response to our bill for $6.00 for a laboratory procedure, determination of Serum Potassium. This procedure is done intermittently on patients receiving diuretic medication for hypertension or cardiac decompensation. The blood is drawn in our office as a convenience to the patient. It is then picked up by an independent laboratory for testing.

The patient's record is taken out of the file, the patient ushered back to the laboratory, the blood drawn and allowed to stand, then contrifuged, with serum removed and packaged for the laboratory. The charge is then entered on the charge slip and patient record and the record returned to the file. The charge slip is then sent down to our bookkeeping department where a ledger is made for the patient, the charge posted and a statement made for the insurance department, where a form is prepared and sent to Wisconsin Medical Assistance requesting payment for this service. A day or two later, when the report comes in from the laboratory, the file is retrieved, the entry made and brought to the attention of the physician ordering the test. He compares it with previous determinations and either sends a card or calls the patient with directions for change or continuation of medications, as indicated. The chart is then refiled. The laboratory charges us $3.00 for their getting the blood, testing it and reporting the results. When payment is made, we again enter, file and post.

It is obvious that 10 cents is an inadequate reimbursement for the work described. The $3.00 handling charge has not seemed to me to be unreasonable. Practices such as ours cannot long endure if this pattern continues.

Thank you for allowing me to share my concern.

Sincerely yours,

James E. Albrecht, MD

* * * * *

Jackson Medical Service Corp.

DECLARATION OF INDEPENDENCE

To All of Our Patients:

Please be advised that as of July 1, 1978 this office will return to the traditional physician/patient relationship common 25 years ago, prior to the evolution of third-party payers.

Since the advent of Medicare in 1968, there has been a steady encroachment on the personal relationship between physicians and patients. That process has accelerated within the last year, culminating with three hundred and ninety plus (390+)

pages of rules recently released, consolidating the federal and state rules and regulations for the Medical Assistance Program. Patients are no longer patients, but "recipients" with numbers — with medical problems also numbered. Physicians are no longer physicians, but rather "providers." More time is expended and more cost incurred in efforts to obtain reimbursement for services rendered than in the actual care of the patient.

Redundant and repetitious filling out of forms, imposed by bureaucracy, has contributed as much as inflation to the ever increasing costs of medical care. Certain conditions require prior approval **before** treatment, **even though** that condition is serious enough in the mind of the patient to have brought him to the office, and serious enough in the mind of the physician to recommend treatment.

We do **not** intend to sign the Medical Assistance Provider Contract in July, and presumptively will not be certified to continue caring for Medical Assistance patients.

Some of the reasons for this action include:

1. Our reluctance to open our patients' records to scrutiny by representatives of the State. We believe these records are personal and privileged.

2. Compliance with 390+ pages of rules subject to change and not compatible with good patient care is impossible.

3. Time spent in paperwork reduces the time and energy available for caring for people.

4. Inconsistent reduction of reimbursement rates while our costs increase due to paperwork in filing reports, deciphering computerized payments lists, crediting partial payments and discounting the balance on both patient charts and ledgers.

5. Third-party payers, with no knowledge of the patient or of the problem treated, set fees retroactively, implying that we have overcharged for services. Then further time is spent answering inquiries as to reasons for our charge.

For these reasons, and more, we will continue, as in the past, the American way of caring for the ill without concern about who pays the bills. We will no longer prostitute our profession, as we have in the past 10 years, by compromising with Medicare and Medical Assistance Planners. This inevitably results in government rules and regulations coming between the physician and patient.

If you do not subscribe to these views, we will continue to care for you until you have arranged for other medical care, and will transfer your records to physicians of your choice.

1. All of our regular patients will continue to be served as in the past and billed as private patients. If you feel our charges unfair, please tell us at the time the service is rendered. If you are unable to pay all or part, please tell us that. Adjustments will be made if necessary.

2. We will accept no new Medical Assistance patients as regular patients, but will render emergency care to those in need, as private patients.

3. Medicaid and Medicare patients and those with private insurance or Blue Shield, will be billed at our usual charge and will be responsible for that charge, regardless of what the Medicaid and Medicare, and private insurer says the charge should be.

This declaration is made with the full knowledge that the consequences may be serious. We feel the consequence of continued cooperation with government planners can lead only to a further erosion of the physician/patient relationship with deleterious effects on both.

James Albrecht, MD, Pres.
Jackson Medical Service Corp.
May 22, 1978

News article, West Bend News, June 1, 1978:

Bureaucracy is too much for Jackson M.D.

By Joan Grosz
News Staff Writer

JACKSON — The latest chunk of bureaucratic red tape to cross Dr. James E. Albrecht's desk here was also the last straw.

It includes a stack of consolidated rules and regs for the state Medical Assistance Program as well as a contract now required of all who provide services to those in the program, which administers Medicaid insurance for some 250,000 recipients in Wisconsin.

Physicians' contracts are due this month. But Dr. Albrecht, head of the Jackson Medical Service Corp., is not going to sign it, he disclosed this week.

That means that as of July 1, he will "accept no new Medical Assistance patients as regular patients, but will render emergency care to those in need, as private patients," according to a letter prepared for all his patients.

And it means that Medicaid won't be picking up the bill for those Medical Assistance patients who decide to stay with him, he said. Rather, they will be billed as private patients and be responsible for their own bills, he said.

Such patients account for eight to 10 percent of the corporation's gross billings, he said. The impact could be "a drastic cut in salaries.

"But it will also mean less paperwork, and we won't have inflated accounts receivable to discount after all that paperwork," including time and effort spent dealing with the state on individual cases, he said.

That is because, he continued, explaining another factor in his haystack of discontent with the program, reimbursements have not kept up with costs.

"They are approximately 75 percent of our usual costs," he said. Thus, while those billings came to approximately $1,200-plus a month, "we've discounted between $300 and $350" each month for the amount not paid by the program.

At the same time, office costs keep rising, he said, noting two people do nothing but handle such paperwork now.

And there is a disparity in reimbursement to physicians, depending on when the doctor entered the program, he said.

Further, he said, the rules and regulations come between the physician and his patient. "We can't practice the one-to-one quality personal care as we had been.

"We're forced to practice almost cookbook medicine; we're told that procedures that we have found have helped our patients are not approved and that we can't be reimbursed for them.

"We will no longer prostitute our profession, as we have in the past 10 years, by compromising with the Medical Assistance Planners," he said in the letter.

It's a matter of principle more than dollars, he indicated. "We're reverting back to the way things were 25 years ago, before the advent of federal insurance programs."

It will again be a private patient-physician relationship, he said. He added that he had already talked with some of those patients who said they understood, but were saddened by the way things have gone.

The action seems in character with the 62-year-old, silver-haired family practitioner who has become something of an institution himself in the 30 years he has practiced here.

For he has taken on government bureaucracy before, scoring some victories, but also losing valuable time and energy he says he would rather spend on practicing medicine.

It does not, however, appear "representative of any large number of physicians in the state," according to Mariellen Kuehn, supervisor of provider relations with the Bureau of

Health Care Financing. That bureau is within the state Department of Health and Social Services, which is responsible for the administration of the Medical Assistance Program.

"The response to the contract from physicians is excellent, really good," she said, noting there are some 9,000 physicians among the 30,000 or so providers of service in the state.

If the experience they have had with other groups from the 50 kinds of providers in the state is any basis, she said, "only about one percent of them appear to be really troubled."

Some of the concern with the contract was expressed by Dr. William Listwan, president of the Washington County Medical society, which has 43 members. It was discussed at a meeting last week, he said.

"No one likes the contract or sees any need for it," he said of the discussion. "It does not benefit the patient or the physician and only adds more rules and regulations to an already inefficient and over-regulated area.

"The wording is unclear to us in many areas; it binds us to rules as of yet not defined and seems an unnecessary piece of paper," he said.

But those at DHSS as well as at the State Medical Society, who have negotiated the interim contract until all the rules and regs are re-consolidated into a "superrule" expected later this year, have tried to reassure the physicians.

"I think the contract is the best possible situation we could have gotten at this time," said Brian Jensen, director of the Physicians alliance Division of the SMS.

"The state has agreed to redo the contract when superrule is finalized," and doctors can decide whether or not to sign the new contract then.

"I think most physicians with a high percent of Medical Assistance patients will sign, whereas those with a fairly insignificant number may feel they can get along with no reimbursement rather than agreeing to a contract they feel is inappropriate," Jensen said.

Jensen had no handle on what would happen among physicians in Washington County, and Listwan said it will be up to individuals whether or not to sign.

Listwan is with the General Clinic of West Bend. Seven of the 11 doctors there are taking new patients, including new Medicaid patients, he said. Those patients account for roughly eight percent of the gross billings, he noted, adding the clinic, too, only gets approximately 75 percent reimbursement for them.

"We don't feel it's right to discriminate against Medicaid patients," he added. But those at the clinic want more information on the contract before making a decision on signing, he said.

There is a rumor another medical group in the county may follow Albrecht's lead, but no similar action has surfaced.

And Don Ryd, director of the Washington County Department of Social Services, hopes none does.

Ryd says 1,547 in the county who get Aid for Families with Dependent Children are eligible for Medical Assistance. So are some 450 who qualify for that assistance only, but not for AFDC. Another 200-plus are in nursing homes, where it supplements their Social Security payments. And still others qualify who get disability payments, but have low income and assets, he said.

"It would be a terrific burden if a significant number of physicians didn't sign, because these people need medical care as much or more than anyone else. If they were excluded as a group, it would create some unfortunate kinds of situations," said Ryd.

"Red tape" is needed to make sure there are proper controls on the use of taxpayer money, Ryd noted. But he said he saw improvement down the line, as a result of current revamping and tightening of the state system for administering Medicaid — despite the added red tape that is distressing physicians like Albrecht.

That is a move that should also make things more equitable as well as increase communication between the providers and the program, says Kuehn.

But Albrecht would like to see things returned to the county level, as they were handled some 12 years ago. He contends county administration would be cheaper, more accountable and more personal.

"I have absolutely no disagreement with Jim Albrecht. I respect him very much as an individual and a physician, and I respect his choice," says Ryd.

"I don't support that happening on a grand scale," Ryd added.

What about Albrecht's patients? Those that stay can still use their Medical Assistance cards for things he might order for them, such as prescriptions or outpatient tests, if the druggists and hospitals are qualified providers, Kuehn said.

As to the rest, it's up to society, Albrecht said, noting society has created the bureaucracy and all its attendant problems.

In fact, burgeoning bureaucracy is one of the reasons for his action now, he said. "I want to raise the question and bring it to the public's attention before it's too late, before proposed national health legislation is in place and the whole situation is much worse, with all the people forced to accept less than the quality health care they have become used to in the past.

"Ever-increasing costs in the science of medicine, resulting in rules and regulations designed to reduce those costs, have inevitably led to the deterioration of the quality of the art of medicine," he added.

But why make a stand now; why not wait at least until superrule is in, as the SMS suggests, since the current contract is said to be no different than the rules that have been in force in the past? In a response that seemed so in character, Albrecht replied by quoting Hamlet's Soliloquy by Shakespeare:

"To be, or not to be: that is the question:
Whether 'tis nobler in the mind to suffer
The slings and arrows of outrageous fortune,
or take arms against a sea of troubles,
and by opposing end them? ..."

* * * * *

June 20, 1978

Mr. Robert W. Kasten, Jr.
Congressman, 9th District
119 Cannon Building
Washington, D.C. 20515

Dear Mr. Kasten:

Thank you for your letter of 6/14/78, as well as your previous letter, which adequately explained my reservations about your use of letterhead of the Congress of the United States in your campaign for Governor.

The copies of letters sent to the Chairman of the 2 House committees were not enclosed in your letter of 6/14/78. I would appreciate receiving them, if possible.

There are several other doctors in our area who have not signed their contract with Medicaid, with more and more rules and clarifications of previous rules coming in the mail, several times a week, it would seem that others, in growing numbers, will follow my lead. In the event that something is not done to curb increasing governmental interference, small practices outside of large groups will be unable to economically survive.

You will be interested in knowing that, without exception, comments from people in all walks of life, from physicians and attorneys to small businessmen, retired people and Medicaid patients, have been uniformly complimentary on my stand. When TV-6 interviewed me a week ago and a short excerpt of the interview was on the 6:00 o'clock news, within 3 or 4 minutes of the completion of the interview, a 58-year-old man, from Milwaukee, called to compliment me on my stand and philosophy and spent about 10 minutes detailing his frustrations with bills dating from December, not paid by Medicare or by his union, private insurance. I am certain that the majority of my patients on Medicare are equally disillusioned with the system. They could be a potent force in alerting the country to the likely ramifications of national health insurance.

Perhaps as Governor you will be able to help make Wisconsin an oasis in the desert of encroaching bureaucracy. You may even be able to instill in the people a sense of pride and self-reliance, that was so common in the Depression days of the '30s. Sunday night, I stopped to visit an old couple who had immigrated from Germany in 1928. They were married in 1930. In 1930 he lost his job. They bought 65¢ worth of material and, between the two of them, hemmed 11 diapers to use on their expected first-born. Last week, I was told of a young welfare recipient who expressed surprise that she was offered an opportunity to learn to do the laundry on diapers, saying that she was allowed $25.00 a month for laundry.

Inflation cannot be licked or the tide stemmed unless more emphasis is put on honest production for dollars received. Federal and State regulations have, over the years, forced small and large business, as well as professional people, to extend ever greater amounts in non-productive record keeping and correspondence, without reimbursement from the governmental unit requiring such records. The ultimate cost can't help but be passed on to the consumer of these goods and services. The paperwork supplied at no direct cost to the governmental units is analyzed, acted on and re-acted on, by ever increasing hordes of State and Federal employees, all in non-productive but extremely costly services.

Thank you for allowing me to ventilate. Best wishes in your campaign.

Sincerely yours,
James E. Albrecht, MD

* * * * *

August 25, 1978

Mr. Donald E. Percy
Secretary
State of Wisconsin
Department of Health and Social Services
1 W. Wilson Street
Madison, WI 53702

Dear Mr. Percy:

Thank you for the courtesy extended Dr. Listwan and myself in inviting us to the meeting at your office on Wednesday. Thank you, too, for your investment of time for our discussion, as well as arranging for Mr. Durkin and Mr. Willkom to participate. I think that we do have a better understanding of each other's problems and, as I told Mr. Ryd on the way back, while we still might be regarded as adversaries, at least we are now friendly adversaries, with both of us understanding some of the problems of the other and, through such understanding, we might even become allies in ameliorating the problems of mutual concern.

I have contacted Terry Willkom, by phone, yesterday with some specific suggestions, particularly relating to some implementation of inter-office contact with providers and your department. Our local hospital administrator, Mr. Bury, had been approached by Dr. Listwan and then by me, independent of each other, with the suggestion that the hospitals might wish to have the same opportunity of one-to-one exchange of problems, as we felt would be beneficial to the physicians. He heartily agrees and would be most receptive to such cooperation. Dr. Zellmer will, in the next few weeks, accumulate definite statistics on their radiological practice, relating to costs of increased paperwork, and will welcome contact by Terry. Dr. Brown, of a large pathology group, feels that somehow or other their business manager, Martin Hofmeister, has solved some of the problems that have plagued most of us, and I suggested to Terry that he contact Dr. Brown or Mr. Hofmeister.

As a result of our conference, I have come to the realization that "even the fleas have fleas" and, perhaps, we can do something to allay each other's itching, caused by federal control. I have asked Carl Zimmerman, of TV-6, to consider contacting you or Mr. Willkom regarding some type of program to acquaint the people with the need for all of us to work together for the good of all.

Please greet Mr. Durkin and Mr. Willkom for me.

Sincerely yours,

James E. Albrecht, MD

* * * * *

August 25, 1978

Mr. Donald Ryd
Director
Washington County Department of Social Services
320 S. 5th Avenue
P.O. Box 476
West Bend, WI 53095

Dear Don:

Thank you very much for taking me to Madison. I thoroughly enjoyed the day and feel it was a good investment of time.

I have been in telephone communications yesterday with Mr. Willkom, with the specific suggestion that, beside implementation of the proposed interchange of personnel between their department and physician's offices, they consider similar discussions and learning of the problems of the hospitals. Mr. Bury welcomed this suggestion and offered to cooperate. In addition, I gave Mr. Willkom the names of physicians who have signed the contract, as well as those who have not, who would be willing to have Mr. Willkom visit their offices to observe specific areas of irritation and potential problems, as well as one officer where, apparently, some of these irritating problems have been solved. It would appear that opening up channels of communication, on a person-to-person basis, will result not only in less animosity, but in a mutual understanding.

The realization that "even the fleas have fleas" could well lead to not only the change from adversaries to friendly adversaries, as I had mentioned to you on the way back from Madison, but perhaps to a status of allies in changing some of the more onerous rules and redundant paperwork imposed on the state and providers by the federal government. As a start, I have called Carl Zimmerman, of Channel 6, suggesting consideration of a program to enlighten the people to the enormity of the problem.

Thank you again.

Sincerely yours,
James E. Albrecht, MD

CHAPTER

32

"Not so Painful, but Enjoyable Interludes"

On this cold January 29, 1993, six months after starting this book, almost eight weeks after Marian's funeral, I realize I am running out of gas. You won, Muriel Kroening, Marty Silseth and John Puotinen.

Marian's stroke occurred eight weeks ago tomorrow. The last several weeks have been so filled with activity, I have had little time to mourn her death or, indeed, rejoice in her life. Preparing this chapter has given me the opportunity to reflect on the many wonderful times Marian and I had with our family, despite my work ethic and rabble-rousing nature.

The last several days have been spent going through the boxes and albums she so meticulously kept. The contents of some of the boxes are now spread out over the dining room table, kitchen counter, den tables and couch, spilling over onto the floor, as I attempt at long last to separate the wheat from the chaff and segregate things which may be of interest to children, nieces and nephews. I marvel anew at how well organized she was in planning jobs to be done or projects to be undertaken.

Among the memorabilia is a photograph taken some months before our marriage, apparently for her graduation picture. As I look at that gentle, trusting smile, realizing the health problems she had up to that point, the poor prognosis given to her by Dr. Helen Dickey, I marvel again at her serenity throughout a much longer life than we had hoped for.

During medical school and internship, no real vacations were possible. In 1949 and subsequently, from time to time we did arrange for coverage of my medical practice for at least a long weekend and usually a week for a vacation to share with my family. For the most part, these were "cheapies," as was our honeymoon. Fishing and sightseeing, occasional swimming and sharing the then still existing roadside inns available for five or six dollars a night provided precious memories.

A few years later, a week-long visit to a house on Lake Metonga in central Wisconsin was enjoyed by Marian's parents with our growing family. This was followed by camping experiences.

Our very first camping experience occurred in 1957, the year following the death of Marian's mother. Grandpa Peters was going through the same sense of loss I am now experiencing. He did not have the outlets to substitute for his grief as I have in completing this book and arranging for a continuation of our partnership, Painter and Potter.

Hopefully, I can arrange for a wide distribution of prints and notecard reproductions of several of her paintings. All of this is with the help of long-time friends, John Miller and Jim Spella, and new friends, Frank DeRaimo, Allan Price and David Rank and other members of the staff of DeRaimo Publishing, Inc. Together, working as a team on earth, under the continuing guidance of our Heavenly Father, may His will be done to achieve the vision He has given for the charitable purposes intended for His glory.

Digression is the story of my life.

Our first camping experience entailed renting an open trailer, trailer hitch and lighting system, along with a tent and other camping equipment, all provided by a service station in Milwaukee. Our trip to the then new Blue Mound State Park, west of Madison, was uneventful. Setting up camp for the first time provided many good laughs as we recalled the events of that and prior vacations.

While we had written directions, as well as verbal directions provided by Mr. Morriaty, who rented us the equipment, putting up the tent for the first time was both a frustrating and hilarious experience. Our first attempts resulted in a total collapse of the tent, completely covering Grandpa Peters. After we extricated him, we read the directions a little more fully and ended up with an acceptable camp: cots and sleeping bags, an Aladdin gas lantern supplementing a beautiful campfire. Our first supper in the "wild" was a delicious stew. Chuck was then three years old, Peter eight and Lynn eleven.

I think we all enjoyed our first night, even though it rained. Early in the morning, the kids were eager to get going. While it still was raining, they were persuaded to stay in bed. With a great deal of difficulty, Grandpa Peters got the charcoal grill lit under an awning and returned to the tent to give Peter an assignment to keep him out of mischief. Even then, communication between adults and children sometimes left something to be desired. A seeming clear direction to put water on the fire for oatmeal was literally interpreted. Grandpa Peters' laborious work to start the fire came to naught as Peter obeyed the command.

We then got dressed and drove to a restaurant in Belmont for a real breakfast instead of our anticipated first campsite breakfast. As I recall, that Sunday breakfast before going to a neighboring church turned out well.

Subsequently, we enjoyed a series of camping trips with a Sears Roebuck tent trailer christened the JaMaLaPaCa — from the first initials of each of our names. Almost every year there would be one or two weekends, as well as the week or ten-day more extensive vacation enjoyed as a family, though sometimes the enjoyment was interspersed with fondly remembered, but less enjoyable at the time, experiences.

We did enjoy trips to the Black Hills in South Dakota, with the experience of almost freezing to death in Cold Water Canyon, visiting Boot Hill and the Passion Play. We enjoyed the wild donkeys and marveled at the presidential heads carved in rock at Mt. Rushmore.

Other camping trips to Yellowstone National Park and the Grand Tetons, as well as into Canada and around Lake Superior are fondly recalled.

On one of our trips to Canada, we were embarrassed when one of our local townspeople, Fritz Held, co-owner of Held's Grocery Store and Meat Market which once stood where the Jackson Post Office now stands, was amazed to find us held up at the border. Canadian border officials were perturbed when I declared that we were going into Canada with, what I admitted was in my drug bag, a few vials of morphine, Demerol and some tablets of Tylenol No. 3, which I habitually carried with me in the event of encountering accidents. I had to deposit the drugs for safekeeping in order to get permission to cross into Canada.

Friends in Jackson got a kick out of hearing how their Doc was stopped at the border. On that trip we came back another way. I never did reclaim my narcotics.

On another trip to Canada we enjoyed productive walleye fishing and our guide's account of the glories of moose hunting. Marian and I did sign up for a fall moose hunting trip.

Friends among our patients offered a variety of big game guns. Never having shot more than a 22 and most often only a BB gun, this was a new experience for both of us. We practiced in a gravel pit near our home and after we got to Canada had further practice under the watchful eye of our Quebecois guide, who spoke very little English.

We didn't get a moose. and never got the promised bear skin rug for which we paid the guide in advance, but we did have a good time.

In 1963, we had the quintessence of all vacations. As the last family vacation before Lynn left home, I had wanted to take the family to Europe. All the kids remonstrated with me that they hadn't seen much of the United States. Our family conference resulted in the agreement that each member of the family would write out what they wanted included in this dream vacation, with the only reservation that it be limited to west of the Mississippi.

Over the course of some weeks, a dream itinerary was developed to the satisfaction of all. We went to AAA to arrange for the incorporation of all the desires of the family into an organized dream vacation — to be accomplished in three weeks. This is a fond remembrance. It was so uncommon that at almost every stop people asked how we enjoyed the things they remember arranging for us several months earlier.

While Marian and I enjoyed the trip, and probably enjoyed it more seeing it through the eyes of our children, I think we were very grateful Chuck was too young to be permitted to take the donkey ride at Yellowstone down into the canyon to the Colorado River. This was especially true after watching the bedraggled veterans of such a trip staggering up the trail.

We often remembered the consternation on the stewardess' face one trip when Peter pointed out in flight that oil was leaking from a wing tank, necessitating our return to Flagstaff, Arizona. Emergency crews had fire equipment all set up and the runway sprayed with a fire retardant when we arrived. We managed to have a safe landing.

Lynn's irritation and embarrassment at her little brother Charles monopolizing the guide who explained how Hoover Dam worked was another fond recollection of that trip.

A trip to Acapulco in 1969, when Pete was in Vietnam and wounded, was an attempt to escape reality. Shorter trips to the American Academy of Family Practice in Colorado, art courses and annual meetings were another change of pace enjoyed by all.

We frequently spoke of the amazement on the faces of our friends, Bill and Margaret Nielsen, and Al and June Grundahl, when they met us at a convention in St. Louis. They asked what route we had taken. It so happened we had decided we wanted to come down along the Mississippi, so we had taken a roundabout way to get to our destination. The usual answer would have been to take a major highway. Our answer, "We took Highway P!"

Two other, more elaborate, vacations by tour, one to Greece and one to northern Europe, provide many enjoyable memories reinforced by albums Marian had assembled. Perhaps the most unique experience was my sitting on the open outdoor privy in Corinth where we fancied St. Paul had relieved himself centuries ago. While they didn't have flush toilets in those days, there was a ditch for running water to carry the excrement away.

The awesome experience of the Alps and the joy of watching flower auctions in Amsterdam are also treasured memories.

A planned tour to the Canadian Rockies never materialized because of an acute medical event while Marian was packing the day before our planned departure. That was the first of several physical problems over the next five years culminating in her death.

Our last vacation, in the middle of November, was an enjoyable trip to the Amana Colonies to pick up a platform rocker we had ordered as a surprise Christmas gift for Lynn. She had admired that chair when she accompanied us on a trip in August. In order to confuse her as to our purpose, we indicated we were going to the medical museum in Prairie du Chien. We did go there on our way home and were surprised to find two pots I had made in the early '80s on display in a glass cupboard, otherwise shared with the memorabilia of more venerable physicians of a bygone generation.

Due to late fishing and duck hunting season, there was "no room in the inn" for fifty miles or more. This was a blessing in disguise, since we so enjoyed our first time ever trip up the west side of the Mississippi. We had a nice overnight stay in a unique bed and breakfast setting, and a trip across the Mississippi and down to return to Prairie du Chien on the east side of the river. We stored the chair at the home of Steve and Kay Chantelois, friends for over thirty years.

Last July, our children, grandchildren, my sister Carol, and long time friend from Colorado, Bob Ditlow, joined us in celebration of Marian's seventieth birthday — a simple dinner party and a tour of Milwaukee Harbor on the Edelweiss sightseeing boat — just the way Marian wished, instead of the grander party I had visualized.

I think she enjoyed a somewhat more ostentatious seventy-fifth birthday I planned for myself. We served over nine hundred and fifty people and gave away more than six hundred and fifty pieces of pottery, and received multiple heart-wrenching tributes of appreciation — and notification that thirty-five charities benefitted from my birthday party. A heartfelt experience, probably of a once-in-a-lifetime caliber, although I did tell everybody to come back for the real party when I am eighty!

I hope this chapter will explain to my readers why we pur-

"Not so Painful, but Enjoyable Interludes"

chased the license plate "WE NJOY" for our family car.

33

"What Does
the Future
Hold?"

None of us has a crystal ball. It is as true now as it was in 1976 when I submitted the article on behalf of the Jackson Medical Service Corporation in the book The History of Jackson, Wisconsin, 1943 to 1976, which has been recently reprinted. That article ends with the paragraph, "What the future holds for Jackson Medical Service, and the continuing history of Jackson, depends upon the inevitable changes that come with burgeoning population and the capacity of the health service personnel to serve the community and *ultimately, the future of any of us in in the hands of God.*"

Even as the family farm as I knew it in my boyhood has disappeared and the one-family farm is close to extinction, even as the dodo became extinct in 1681, so is it likely the single family practice will soon become extinct.

Webster's Third New International Dictionary, unabridged, copyright 1961, clearly offers this additional definition for a dodo: "A person who is simplemindedly unaware of changing conditions and new ideas; a dull, stupid person."

Perhaps I qualify. I have long felt, as John must have felt two hundred centuries ago, that I was a "lone voice crying in the wilderness." In the mid-1960s, when Medicare was being proposed in Congress, I remember writing to our then Senator Alexander Wiley, prognosticating exactly what was going to happen. The government interposed itself between patient and physician with rules and regulations. The inevitable result of that action has had an adverse impact on patients, physicians and society as a whole.

At the risk of being considered in the second category of the definition of the dodo, I am entering a copy of a June 21, 1991 letter addressed to President Bush with the hope that at least some of the suggestions made then might still be considered at the national level as the Clinton Administration is wresting with the product of long-term neglect and mismanagement.

Dear President Bush:

This letter is addressed to you. Copies are being sent to all members of your Cabinet as well as to members of Congress in the hope that the thoughts of a 75-year-old family physician in practice since 1948 might help in dealing with the ever increasing cost of health care.

A few weeks ago our pharmacist, Mel Esselman, told me of a 15% increase after an 8% increase six months earlier in the cost of two currently popular and effective antihypertensives, Capoten and Corgard. Other pharmaceutical companies have increased prices at an annual rate of 6 to 22%. Due to recent Federal OBRA rebates, additional increases are anticipated. Despite ongoing efforts to control costs and still maintain patient care, pharmacists are forced to pass, on some of these increases. This week one of my long time patients, Carl Wegner Sr., informed me he had cut his Corgard to one-half of the prescribed dose to reduce his cost to a level he could afford. Other patients have been non-compliant when faced with the choice of having money for food and shelter and other family needs or preserving their physical well being.

Physicians and hospitals often have been accused of being responsible for the escalating costs of health care. Some of this criticism is valid. Other factors including actions of government over the years are equally to blame.

Some years ago costs of medical education doubled because the interest on money borrowed to finance education was no longer considered a tax deduction in contrast to an equal amount invested in a business: As a consequence medical students by the time they have finished medical school and 3 years or more of residency have borrowed a large amount on which interest has compounded: One young doctor I know borrowed $70,000 to finance his education. By the time he became employed by our clinic that $70,000 compounded quarterly had reached $140,000: Interest payments, which are not tax deductible, continue to be a terrific burden. The State and Federal Departments of Revenue get 25-30% of current income; with the need to repay on principal and regular monthly interest, he has little to meet house payments and support his wife and children. How long he can exist and get out of debt is anyone's guess.

Could this be the reason 55% of Phd degrees awarded in the United States go to foreign graduates as reported in the last few months on CNN?

Times have changed: When I finished medical school and internship and started practice I owed my mother something like $6,000: At $2.00 an office call and $4.00 home calls and 75¢ a mile, it took about 10 years to repay my loan, even with the benefit of interest payments being tax deductible at that time.

Currently clinics are competing to attract a too small number of primary care physicians to meet the needs of their communities. Many rural communities can't afford to attract physicians to serve their need. Most physicians can't afford to move to physician poor areas even if subsidized. No matter how idealistic one is, the harsh realities demand attention to self preservation.

Another great concern is that young physicians caring for Medicare patients are paid less than adequately, 20% less than experienced physicians: Additionally clinics have increased costs in administrating variable fee schedules.

Medicare has not kept up with inflationary costs of care, resulting in the cost shift to all non-Medicare patients.

It appears the only organizations having reasonable security are the insurance and pharmaceutical companies.

Another significant item is the tendency to try to preserve life long beyond the time an individual ceases to be productive in any way and would rather be dead than to burden his or her family and society for a few more years of meaningless existence.

We were born to live, produce, reproduce and die. Today it seems the equation has changed to do as little as we can to get by: Earn by fair means or foul enough to finance a life of leisure and enjoyment at an early retirement age.

Today I had to suggest to 94-year-old Herb Mueller that it would be well to ask his nephew to cut the lower limbs off the trees on the two acre lawn he cuts with a riding lawn mower so that he doesn't injury himself seriously while continuing to duck under the branches, scratching his head and arms. *His is a meaningful life.*

The lives of countless people in nursing homes are preserved indefinitely to no end. We are postponing death - not increasing life.

My hope is that you and Mrs. Bush may continue to be productive as long as God wills it, and that in His Grace he sees fit to take you to Him before you reach a vegetative existence.

It would be my suggestion that you convene experienced family physicians, perhaps 2 or 3 from each state, to work with members of Congress in a cooperative non-adversary manner to solve some of the problems of concern to so many.

Thank you and all others receiving this letter for your patience in reading this lengthy epistle. Please give it your prayerful attention.

Sincerely yours,
James E. Albrecht, MD

While our nation and the international community, as well as society as a whole, have reached the point of a person up to his neck in quicksand, I still believe that if we put our reliance on God, with His help, all things are possible.

It is my prayer that the current Administration will see fit to enlist the support of God as they attempt to lead this country to the Promised Land. Amen.

Epilogue
Meet My Friend,
Jesus Christ
(Layman's sermon,
Christ Lutheran Church,
June 22, 1986)

"**E**xcept you become as little children you shall not enter the Kingdom of Heaven." It is for that reason that I tell my story as one child to all you other children of our Heavenly Father.

Two weeks ago, in mini-Sunday School, ACTS (Active Christian Teen Students, a youth group) presented a skit following which we were asked to share our experiences of when we felt unwanted and out of the mainstream. This morning, I will share with you some of the experiences of my three score and ten years which have influenced my life and helped me to answer the question Jesus asked of his Disciples, "Who do you say that I am, Jimmy Albrecht?"

He asks that question of each of us, and upon our answer depends our very life here on earth and in Heaven to come. Each of us, according to Kahlil Gibran, "stands alone in the knowledge of God and in his own knowledge of God and his understanding of the earth." We come to that knowledge of God from personal experience and from interrelationships with others. Some of us have earthshaking experiences, some more quiet and reflective pathways to God. Daily contact with God in prayer and meditation are a necessity if we are not to make too many detours!

When Phillip asked the Ethiopian eunuch whether he understood the Scripture he was reading, the answer was, "How can I understand except that some man should guide me?" Guidance comes from listening to sermons, attending Sunday School, sharing in discussion with fellow Christians, reading of the Scriptures and good books. The intermingling of all these things shapes our lives for better or for worse. Our past, our present, and our future completely depend on our answer to the questions, "Who do you say that I am?" and "How do you say that I am?" May the Holy Spirit enter our hearts and minds to lead us on the right pathway in life.

In answer to the question, a disciple asked, "Sir, why are you going to reveal yourself only to us disciples and not to the world at large?" Jesus replied, "Because I will only reveal myself to those who *love* me and *obey* me. The Father will love them too and will come to them and live with them. Anyone who doesn't obey me doesn't love me. Remember, I am not making up this answer to your question. It is the answer given by the Father who sent me. I am telling you these things now while I am still with you, but when the Father sends a comforter instead of me, and by a comforter I mean the Holy Spirit, he will teach you much, as well as remind you of everything that I myself have told you."

God works in mysterious ways to shape our lives. All of us

have had experiences that we would rather not have, only to find, as time goes on, that we look at them as blessings that have helped us grow closer to God.

A potter at his wheel, creating a piece of art from a lump of clay, needs to exert pressure on that clay first to center it, then to open it and then form it. Without the friction of his hands and the guidance of his mind, the clay becomes waste and not a beautiful vase or a useful bowl. Just so, God exerts pressure on our lives to form us into the men and women He would have us to be. Certainly, my life has been influenced both directly and indirectly by contact with many people through the years, and I will share some of this with you.

Like Timothy, I was fortunate enough to have a mother and grandmother who taught me to pray. Even now, when I take my 94-year-old mother out to dinner, she prays before we eat: "Come, Lord Jesus, be our guest and let these gifts to us be blessed." As a boy, I remember fantasizing that Jesus was going to make an appearance at our table. I wonder if any of the younger children still have that thought?

I don't remember my baptism, which occurred at about two months of age, but I do remember three years of Confirmation school with Pastor Gammerlien teaching the catechism as well as demonstrating his knowledge of Greek. I remember the games of marbles and mumbletypeg at recess, and also remember the anxieties the Sunday before Confirmation when, in front of the Church, we confirmands had to answer questions. Confirmation Day in 1929 made me a confirmed member of the Church. At that point, I had no real appreciation or personal knowledge of the Lord Jesus Christ. I had learned about Him and about His Church, but I hadn't gotten to *know* and to *love* Him.

In 1932, when my father had a farm accident, I became a school dropout and was forced to run the farm to support our family during the Depression. Those were frustrating times.

Looking back, good came of evil, because during that four-year period I became acquainted with and developed a friendship with Dr. E. M. Keller, an osteopathic physician and a dedicated Methodist layman. He introduced me to philosophy and books, among which was Lloyd C. Douglas' *Magnificent Obsession*, and for the first time I had a realization of the person of Jesus Christ in my own life. "Whatsoever you shall ask in My name with a believing heart that will I give unto you."

Contact with other denominations enlarged my concepts beyond what I then considered a rather stuffy Lutheran Doctrine.

The ecumenical experience that spread over the next several years led to my conviction that if the United States ever got into war I would be unable to bear arms. With Japan's invasion of China and then in 1939 Germany's invasion of Poland, it became more and more likely that those convictions would be getting me into trouble. I was able to return to high school in 1936 and on to the University in 1937. A lot of questions were raised in my mind when my father killed himself in 1938 out of frustration and depression over his crippled body.

At about that time, I had the good fortune of meeting the second man to shape my life, Dr. Morris Wee of Bethel Lutheran Church in Madison. In 1939 when it came time to register for the draft, I registered as a conscientious objector and had quite a few confrontations with the draft board which wanted me to stay in medical school and promised never to draft me if only I would withdraw my statement of belief from their files. That was one of the times I didn't share with ACTS at mini-Sunday School a few weeks ago. I had a sense of loneliness because family and friends, for the most part, didn't understand. I felt something like Luther: "I can do no other, so help me God." Jesus did help me with a sense of personal presence. That led to another blessing, being inducted into "work of national importance" in a conscientious objector camp run by the Quaker's American Friends Service Committee at Merom,

Indiana. Here I came in contact with like-minded individuals from many different denominations. I was in correspondence with many of the only seventeen other Lutherans in the United States who were conscientious objectors in the months before Pearl Harbor. When we speak of minorities, *we were* a minority in the Lutheran Church. Beside Jesus being my friend, Pastor Morris Wee and the people of Bethel Lutheran Church continued to accept me as one of their own. The camp at Merom was designed to provide for soil conservation, but I was kept in camp as a cook and also worked in personnel. Somewhat later, I was transferred to Cleveland State Hospital where I observed that chaplains were apparently of more help to the patients than the doctors and attendants were.

Another disheartening experience occurred in 1943: After deciding that I could accept noncombat status in the Armed Services, I was briefly in the Navy, only to have a psychiatrist put a big "U" on my chest and back meaning "unfit for good military material." When I went to the chaplain, he said, "Albrecht, you go back to Madison and tell Morris Wee I am ashamed that a man with your ideas should be a member of the Norwegian Lutheran Church." It helped a bit when I asked if he was speaking as a commander in the United States Navy or as a Man of God, and ultimately he apologized when he heard a little more of my story. My discharge read, "Too inelastic for good military material."

There was another period of farming and on January 1, 1944, I had my first date with Marian. We married on August 18, 1944, putting our lives in God's hands. I returned to medical school on January 1, 1945, and subsequently found that I had a tuberculous spot on my right lung. This was apparently contracted during my work as lab technician at Cleveland State Hospital as a CO. Our prayers were answered, and it healed without my having to quit medical school.

He has been with us ever since. In sickness and in health,

we have endured and have grown closer to Him.

In the Second Lesson of the Day we heard, "And if you are in Christ then you are Abraham's offspring, heirs according to promise, "You will recall that God told Abraham, after the death of his father, "Leave your own country behind you and your own people and go to the land I will guide you to. If you do, I will cause you to become the father of a great nation. I will bless you and make your name famous and you will be a blessing to many others. I will bless those who bless you and curse those who curse you and the entire world will be blessed because of you."

God expects something in return for his blessings. In the Book of James we are told, "You will be judged on whether or not you are doing what Christ wants you to do, so watch what you do and what you think, for there will be no mercy to those who have shown no mercy, but if you have been merciful then God's mercy toward you will win out over his judgement against you." (*The Living Bible Paraphrased*, Tyndale.)

Dear Brothers, what is the use of saying that you have faith and are Christians if you aren't proving it by helping others? Will that kind of faith save anyone? If you have a friend who is in need of food and clothing and you say to him, "Well, good bye and God bless you, stay warm and eat hearty," then don't give him clothes or food. What good does that do? So you see, it isn't enough just to have faith. You must also do good because you have faith. Faith that doesn't show itself by Christian action is no faith at all, it is dead and useless. "Christ has no hands but our hands to do the work that must be done." Christ tells us in John 15:14, "Ye are my friends if you do whatsoever I command you". In answering the question of the scribe or lawyer, "Which is the great Commandment of Law," Jesus said, "Thou shalt love the Lord thy God with all thy heart and with all thy soul and with all thy mind." This is the first and greatest Commandment. The Second Commandment is like unto it, "Thou shalt love thy neighbor as thyself." In these two Commandments hang all the laws of the prophets.

Jesus asks us the pointed question, "Why do you call me Lord, Lord, and do not the things which I say?" He also tells us, "Not everyone that sayeth Lord, Lord shall enter into the Kingdom of God but he that doeth the will of my Father in Heaven."

It is my firm conviction, based on my own experience and the experiences of many others, that He expects us to be liberal with what He has given us. As we share with others in His name, there will be more to share. Our cup will continue to overflow if we don't try to keep it all for ourselves. We have been blessed to be a blessing.

Let us reflect on the words of wisdom in the last Chapter of Ecclesiastes: "Let us hear the conclusion of the whole matter, fear God and keep His Commandments for this is the whole duty of man. God shall bring every work into judgment with every secret thing whether it be good or whether it be evil."

In conclusion, it is my prayer that we may all experience the love, companionship and guidance of our Friend, Savior and Commander-In-Chief, Jesus Christ.

Amen.

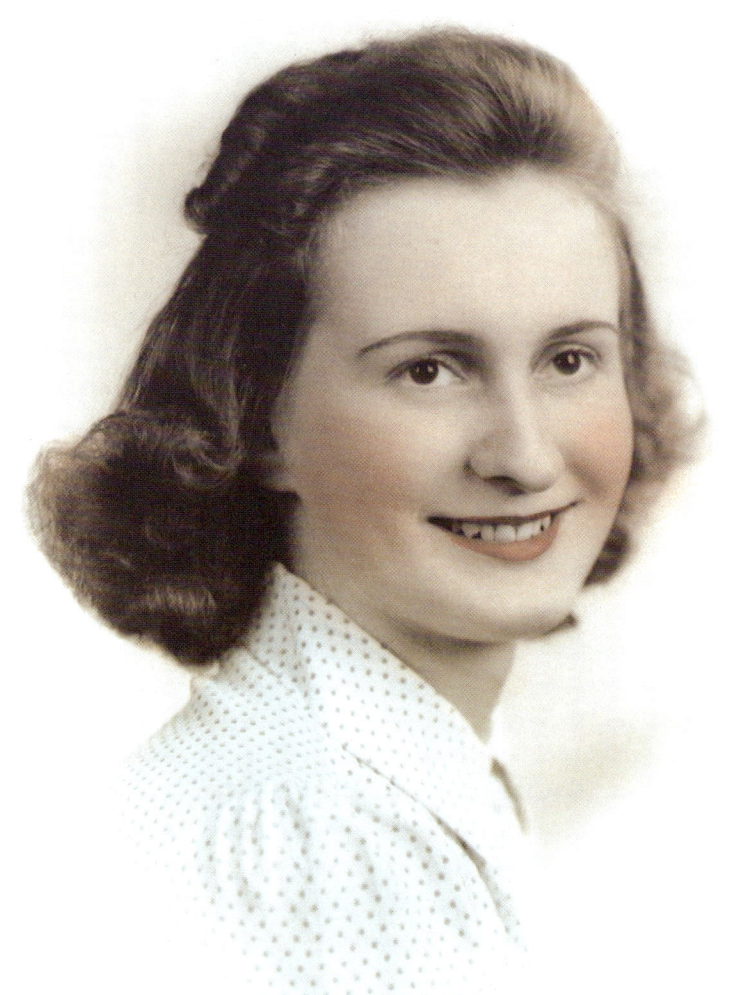

The girl that
I married

Marian's Section

A credo we lived by written on birch bark.

Let there be spaces
in your togetherness
And let the winds
of the heavens dance
between you.
— KAHLIL GIBRAN

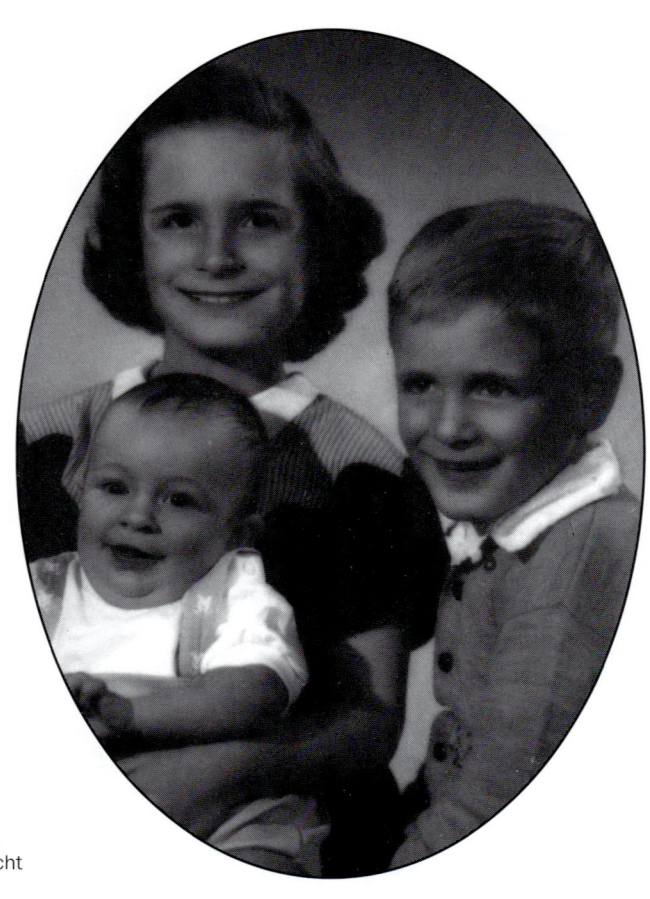

Right: Lynn, Peter, and Charles Albrecht about 1953.

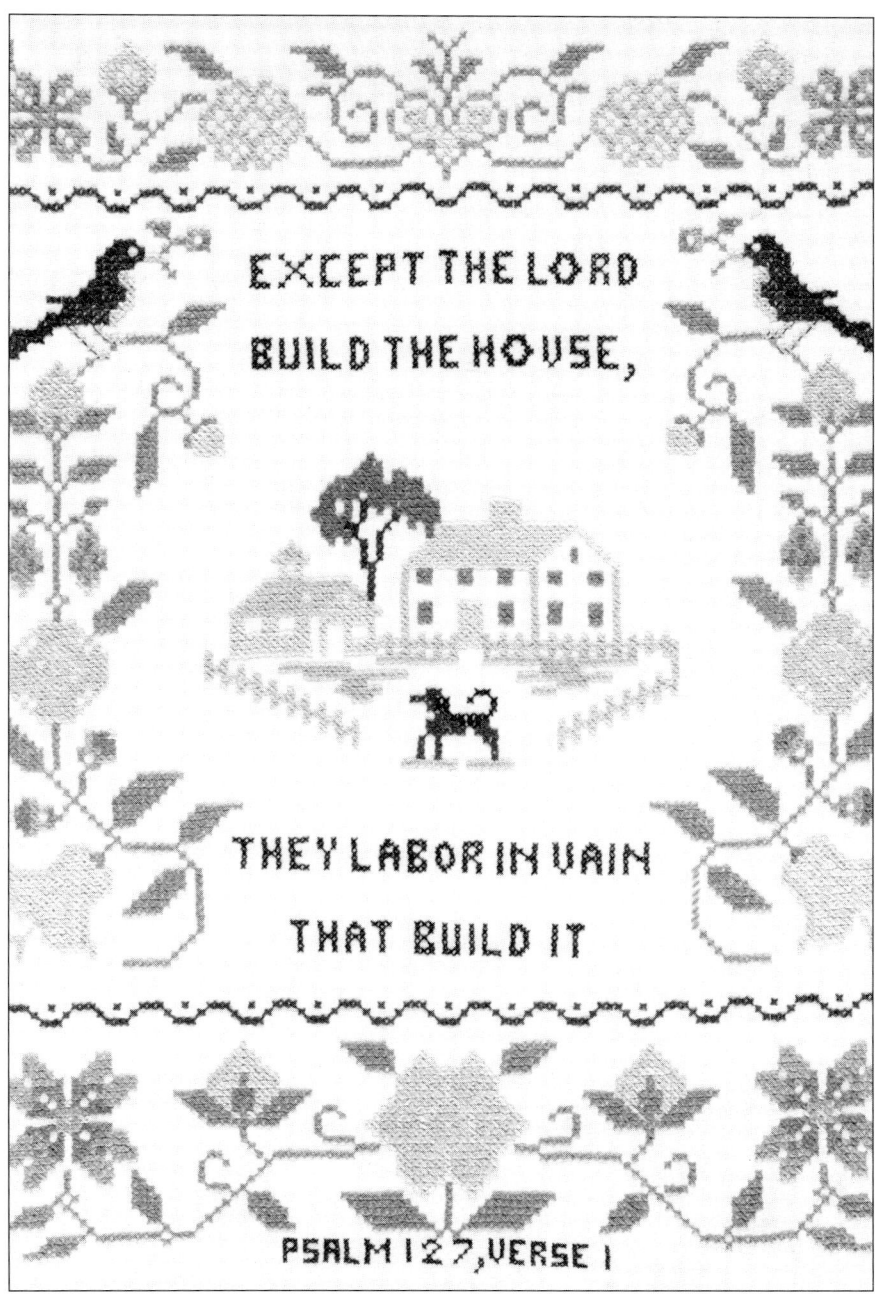

EXCEPT THE LORD BUILD THE HOUSE,

THEY LABOR IN VAIN THAT BUILD IT

PSALM 127, VERSE 1

Done by Marian during the nine months we waited for our house to be built in 1956.

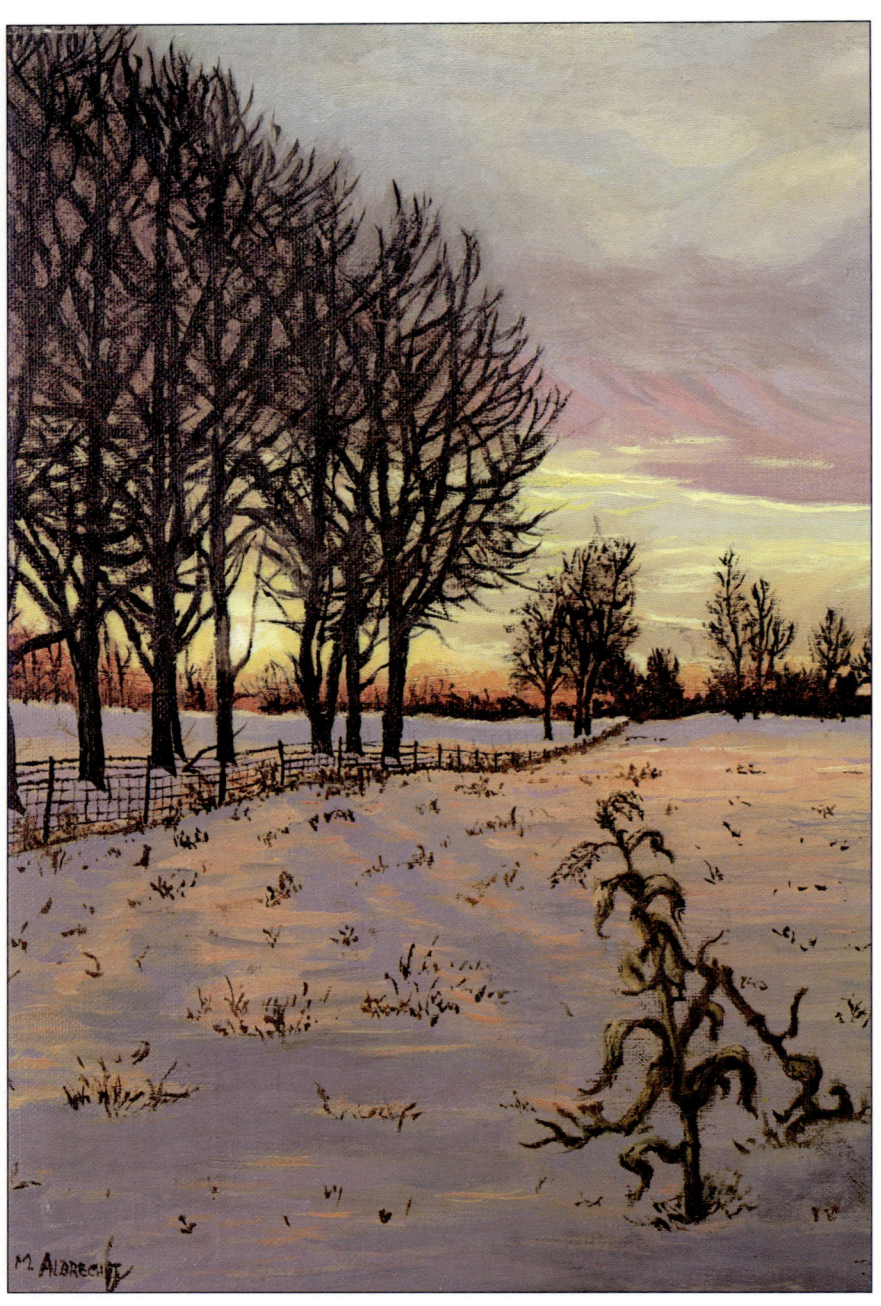

Wintery sunset.

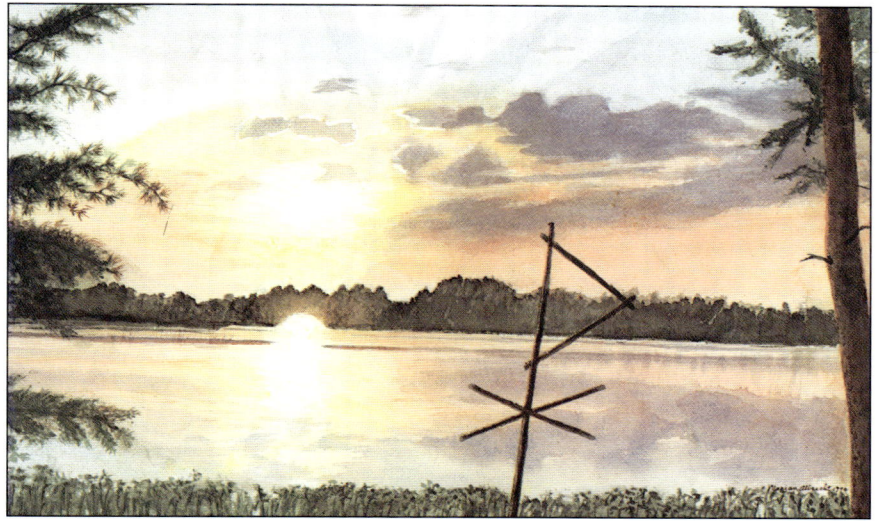

Waypost Chi Rho.

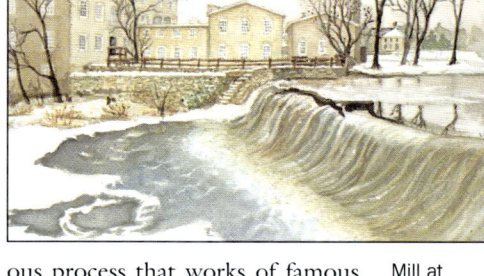

Mill at Cedarburg, Wisconsin

Art and music were Marian Albrecht's avocation; she shared much of her work readily with others. Though not formally trained, she reached a level of competency in sketching that made her landscapes, particularly, a pleasure to look at. But even more important, much of her work had a quality that touched people. They reacted. She worked in many types of media but preferred watercolor, by no means the easiest to execute.

Upon her death, December 7, 1992, many of her friends asked her husband, Jim, for reproductions of some of their favorite paintings. He not only agreed but made arrangements to have prints made by one of the leading area printers for high-quality art reproductions. Marian's pieces will follow the same fastidi-

ous process that works of famous professionals are put through. Materials of archival quality will be used. Proofs will be painstakingly studied for strict adherence to the original. We can do no more.

These are limited editions; all prints will be numbered with Marian's signature and Jim's authorizing initials (standard procedure in the art world for a deceased artist). About May 31, prints will be available at locations yet to be announced. All reproductions are

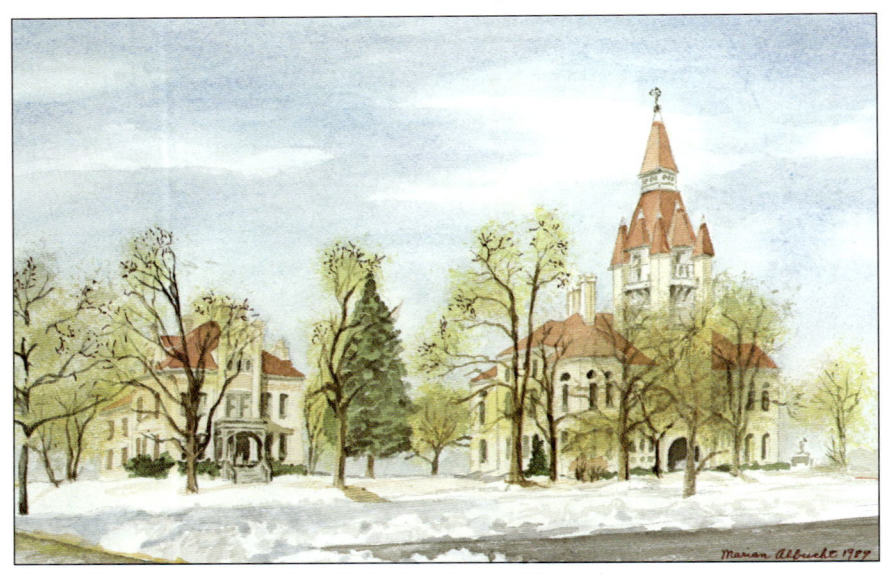

Above: Old courthouse and jail in Washington County, Wisconsin.

from watercolor originals except Wintery Sunset, which is reproduced from an oil painting.

Net proceeds (after production costs have been recovered) from two of the prints will go to organizations that were of particular interest to the artist. Revenue from the Old Washington County Courthouse and Jail will benefit the Washington County Historical Society and Waypost Chi Rho proceeds will go to Crossways Lutheran Camping Ministries.

Bottom: Around a bend on a canoe trip down the Plover River in Wisconsin.

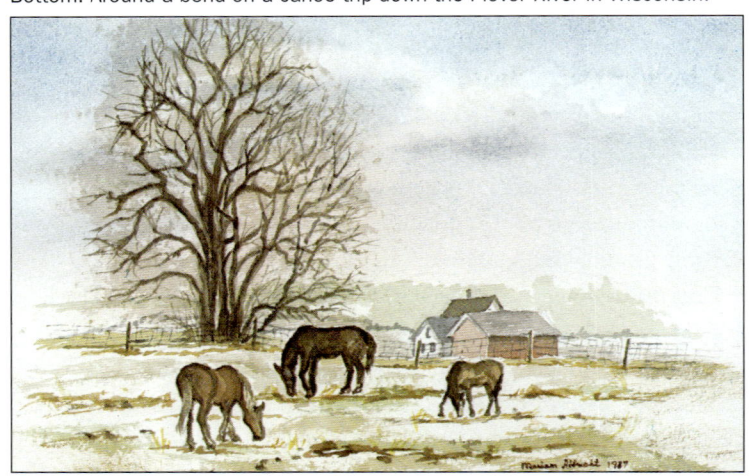

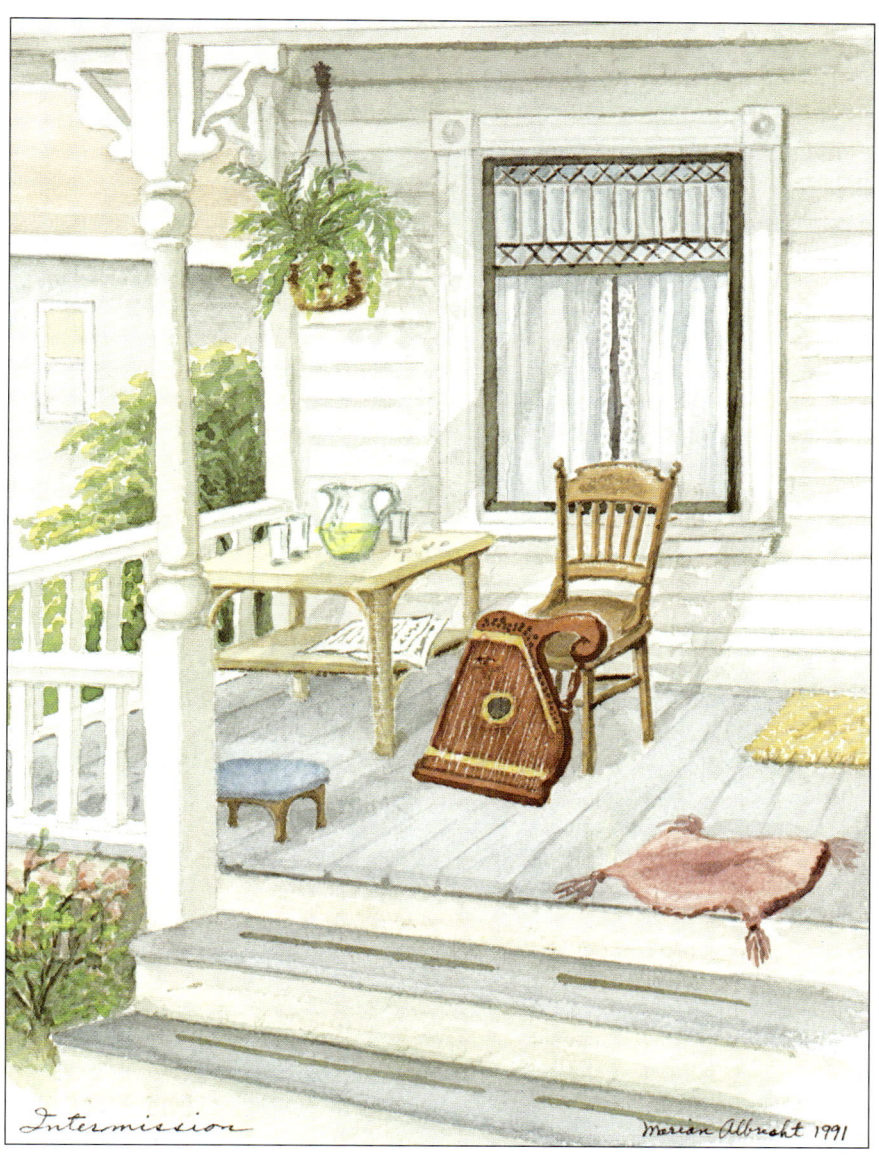

"Intermission".

ORDER FORM
(Please copy or cut on dashed lines and send with remittance.)

Please send me:

Number Ordered	Item	Cost Each	Cost Subtotal
_____	Old courthouse and jail in Washington County, Wisconsin.	$ 40.00	_____
_____	Around a bend on a canoe trip down the Plover River in Wisconsin.	$ 35.00	_____
_____	Waypost Chi Rho.	$ 40.00	_____
_____	"Intermission"	$ 40.00	_____
_____	Mill at Cedarburg, Wisconsin.	$ 35.00	_____
_____	Wintery sunset.	$ 35.00	_____
_____	"The Life And Times Of A Country Doctor"	*$ 23.45	_____
_____	ORDER TOTAL		_____

* $19.95 + $1.00 tax + $2.50 shipping

Please print or write carefully. -

Name: _____

Address: _____

City: _____ State: _____ ZIP: _____

Telephone: _____

Please mail with remittance to:

Jim Albrecht
2487 Pleasant Valley Road
Jackson, WI 53037